Living & Loving

The Marathon of Life

Experiencing the
Electricity of Life

Lisa M. Harper
www.marathonmission.net
lisa@marathonmission.net

VerticalView Publishing

Living and Loving – The Marathon of Life
By Lisa M. Harper
Copyright © 2009 Lisa M. Harper
Reprinted 2013

ISBN 13: 978-0-9823356-0-4
ISBN 10: 0-9823356-0-1
Library of Congress Control Number: 2009923134

Cover and book design: Nick Zelinger, NZ Graphics
www.nzgraphics.com

Editing: Dan Van Veen
Author photos: Katie Kieft
Marathon Mission photos: Tom Martindale and Jeff Kindy

Published by VerticalView Publishing
PO Box 262, Clare, MI 48617
Phone: 734-775-3073
www.verticalviewpublishing.com
Email: lisa@marathonmission.net

This book is available at www.marathonmission.net,
www.themarathonoflife.com, www.verticalviewpublishing.com,
and www.lisaharpermarathonmom.com.
Also available at online retailers including Amazon.com.

Printed in the United States of America
First Edition 2009
Reprinted 2013

"You've all been to the stadium
and seen the athletes race.
Everyone runs; one wins. Run to win.
All good athletes train hard.
They do it for a gold medal
that tarnishes and fades.
You're after one that's gold eternally."

(The Message)

This book is dedicated to the Lord who has given me this opportunity. To Scott, my husband. You are the man I respect most in this life. You continually fan into flame the dreams within me. To my children: Autumn, Jonathan, Victoria, and Jasmine. You provide me with endless joy and are precious jewels in my crown. Together we experience the electricity of life!

CONTENTS

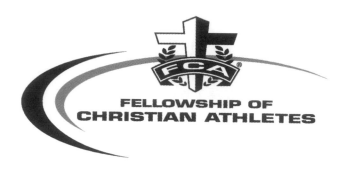

IMPACTING THE WORLD FOR CHRIST
THROUGH SPORTS

Since 1954, the Fellowship of Christian Athletes has challenged athletes and coaches to impact the world for Jesus Christ. FCA is cultivating Christian principles in local communities nationwide by encouraging, equipping and empowering others to serve as examples and to make a difference. Reaching over 1.7 million people annually on the professional, college, high school, junior high and youth levels, FCA has grown into the largest interdenominational sports ministry in the world. Through FCA's "4 C's" of Ministry: Coaches, Campus, Camps and Community and the shared passion for athletics and faith, lives are changed for current and future generations.

VISION
To see the world impacted for Jesus Christ
Through the influence of athletes and coaches

MISSION
To present to athletes and coaches and all whom they influence,
the challenge and adventure of receiving Jesus Christ as Savior and Lord,
Serving Him in their relationships and in the fellowship of the church.

VALUES
Integrity – Serving – Teamwork - Excellence

* Maurie Holbrook / FCA Northern Michigan / mholbrook@fca.org

INTRODUCTION

"*I* want to be a writer!*" For over 30 years I have hidden this dream in my heart, not knowing if it would ever come true. I write this book now because I believe it is a message worth writing and reading. Life truly is like a marathon. There are highs and lows. There are valleys and mountaintops. There is even a start and a finish.

Think about these stages of your marathon of life: inspiration, preparation, perspiration, initiation, continuation, obstruction, anticipation, and celebration.

In *Living and Loving – The Marathon of Life*, I have tried to include a variety of real life experiences as they relate to these areas. My hope is that you can see yourself in some of them as well. How would you respond? What would you do differently? What truths can you take with you?

No matter where you are in life, reading *Living and Loving – The Marathon of Life* will give you opportunities to reflect on your journey and even improve certain aspects that may have been nagging you for a while.

I trust that this book will be friendly, warm and conversational. While writing each story, I pictured myself talking to you face to face. Those of you who know me well are aware that I am a positive person by nature. Although some kind of pep talk comes out on every page, I was not bashful in letting you see some of my shortcomings, too. Hopefully you will sense from me a genuine respect and connection with you, along with a dash of humor along the way. You may even get a little kick in the pants without knowing it!

"Employ your time in improving yourself by other men's writings so that you shall come easily by what others have labored hard for."
~ Socrates

While there is a deliberate sequence of stages as they relate to the marathon of life, feel free to pick up *Living and Loving* and randomly read any chapter. The first chapter in each of the eight stages refers to running in some way. The remaining chapters in each stage relate to all sorts of everyday topics of interest. Whether you read this book straight through or just glance at it for five minutes, your day will be brighter for it.

Finally, my intention is that you will be motivated and encouraged by the words on these pages. As a result, through taking small, significant, intentional strides, you'll improve your marathon of life by *Living and Loving*, one step at a time!

"Every day you may make progress.
Every step may be fruitful. Yet there will
stretch out before you an ever-lengthening,
ever ascending, ever-improving path.
This adds to the joy and glory of the climb."
~ Winston Churchill

STAGE 1

Inspiration

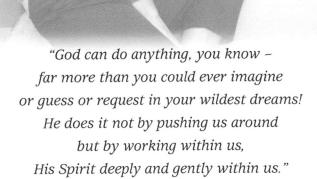

"God can do anything, you know –
far more than you could ever imagine
or guess or request in your wildest dreams!
He does it not by pushing us around
but by working within us,
His Spirit deeply and gently within us."

(The Message)

A Hobby a Day

"A hobby a day keeps the doldrums away."
~ Philis McGinley

W hat's your favorite hobby? What inspired you to start it? What motivates you to continue?

Running is definitely one of my passions, but it has not always been. My adolescent sport was gymnastics, consisting of time on the balance beam, uneven parallel bars, vault and floor exercise. Sit-ups and push-ups were my bread and butter. In fact, I believed that if my muscles weren't reasonably sore the day after a workout, then I didn't work them out enough! As a result, I challenged my muscles for years.

"The last three or four reps is what makes the muscle grow. This area of pain divides the champion from someone else who is not a champion. That's what most people lack… having the guts to go on and just say they'll go through the pain no matter what happens."
~ Arnold Schwarzenegger

Have you ever started to work on a goal, only to abandon it within days? Two weeks…that's all I lasted on the school track team. As a teenager, the only running

I would do was down the runway towards the gymnastics vault. As for distance runners, I felt sorry for them. They looked so skinny and emaciated. Where were the "healthy-looking" bulging muscles that I was used to seeing among gymnasts?

"Great ideas originate in the muscles."
~ Thomas Alva Edison

Can you identify a specific, positive event that changed your life forever? For me, once I set foot on the campus of Oral Roberts University in Tulsa, Oklahoma, my whole-person philosophy of life really flourished! Not only were we required to strengthen our minds and our spirits, but we also completed a field test (running, walking or biking) every semester. What? Those sports were a far cry from doing the splits or standing on my hands, but I loved the aerobic challenge. Have you been energized by a physical feat?

As the weeks went on I decided to run another lap, and another, and another.

"Constant repetition carries conviction."
~ Robert Collier

Within three months of running I ran 6 miles at a time. At age 18, thirty-mile weeks were common for me. Unfortunately, I was clueless as to the proper shoes to wear, thereby taping my arches with masking tape for optimum support. Aren't tennis shoes good enough for running? No, sir! Tennis shoes are meant for *tennis*, not running! With inspiration (and ignorance) I increased my running regime.

> *"When people wear shoes that don't fit them,*
> *it says something about their soul.*
> *Generally, I think it means*
> *they are good people."*
> ~ William Thorton

What inspired me to continue running? I discovered that God gave me physical endurance, and I was intrigued to push it to the limit. For 10 years I had spent the bulk of my athletic career inside a gym. With running, I was able to experience nature and its Creator in a whole new way. I had no idea where running would take me, but it was a new love that I wanted to foster. I felt close to God while running and even memorized Proverbs (from note cards) on my daily jaunts. (Those were some sweaty note cards!) This life-style approach to strengthening my body, mind, and spirit made more sense to me than ever before. It's who I am today.

> *"When I run, I feel God's pleasure."*
> ~ Eric Liddell

What (or who) inspires you to be healthy in body, mind, and spirit? Picture the person you want to be. What steps are you taking to get there?

Somewhere over the Rainbow

The most humbling of all occupations in the world is that of being a parent. (Even a restroom janitor will know that when he's done his job well, the final product will surely shine! With parenting, we sow good seeds and hope for the best!) I used to think I knew most of life's answers until our four children were added to the Harper mix. Then I became woefully aware of my inadequacies and need for divine assistance. My husband, Scott, would second the motion.

*"If nature had arranged that husbands
and wives should have children alternatively,
there would never be more than three in a family."*
~ Lawrence Housman

Which family members inspire you? Your Sister Susie, Daughter Daisy, Son Simon or Uncle Arthur may not be perfect, but being created in God's image, there is some good in all of them. As a parent, I have been inspired by the uniqueness of each one of our children.

Throughout the ages, personalities have often been characterized into four categories. (Which one describes you? Visit www.ylcf.org to learn more.) Experts suggest that we are born with one predominant personality type, with various degrees of others. Hippocrates used the words Choleric, Sanguine, Phlegmatic, and Melancholy to describe individualities. Artistic philosophers might refer to them as Green, Orange, Blue, and Gold. In children's literature this would be Rabbit, Tigger, Pooh, and Eeyore. As Charlie Brown characters, these are Lucy, Snoopy, Charlie Brown, and Linus. I like to think of my four children along the lines of Dr. Gary Smalley's analogy: Lion, Otter, Golden Retriever, and Beaver.

Our Lion (with Golden Retriever tendencies as well) is Autumn. As the oldest of four, she is direct, self-propelled, administrative, and a powerful leader. Autumn displays the defensive skills of a lawyer along with the compassionate ways of Mother Teresa…particularly where the needy are concerned.

"I am sometimes a fox and sometimes a lion.
The whole secret of government lies in
knowing when to be one or the other."
~ Napoleon Bonaparte

Our Otter is Jasmine. As a spirited, active, expressive young lady, she sure knows how to put on a show. "Jazzy" already writes romantic poems and can swing dance her way into anyone's heart. Moreover, her knack for mothering younger children would put many of us to shame.

"Are you upset little friend? Have you been lying awake worrying? Well, don't worry...I'm here. The flood waters will recede, the famine will end, the sun will shine tomorrow, and I will always be here to take care of you."
~ Charlie Brown to Snoopy

Jonathan is our Golden Retriever. He's solid, considerate, amiable, and steady. Every family needs at least one innovative, generous, peaceful, and dependable brother to protect his sisters!

"He is your friend, your partner, your defender.
He will be yours, faithful and true,
to the last beat of his heart. You owe it to him
to be worthy of such devotion."
~ Unknown

Leave it to Beaver. When the Harpers need a task to be tackled, we call on Victoria. Her systematic, economic, high-quality ways inspire her to live with excellence. Adults recruit Victoria to do what they can't do, or don't have the compliant perseverance to finish, in their race of life! Go, Victoria!

"Be studious in your profession, and you
will be learned. Be industrious and frugal,

and you will be rich. Be sober and temper-
ate, you will be healthy. Be in general,
virtuous, and you will be happy."
~ Benjamin Franklin

What colors of the rainbow make up your family?
What tint are you? Knowing your temperament and
those around you is one of life's greatest opportunities!

Heed the Call

"What should I do with my life?" That's the million-dollar question. Sometimes we have been forced to take any job that's available to us, but if we are fortunate in life, we will also have those moments when we are truly "flowing in our gifts."

"Everybody has talent, it's just a matter
of moving around until you've
discovered what it is."
~ George Lucas

What are your strong points? What skills come easily to you? Initially your own strengths may be difficult for you to realize, because you are just "being who you are."

"This is how I define talent;
it is a gift that God has given us in secret,
which we reveal without knowing it."
~ Charles De Montesquieu

I found this quote to be true when I was trying to decide on a profession. I basically love life and embrace the best parts of the arts, sciences, history, culture, family, service, and faith. I want to use whatever talents I have to make a difference in this world.

*"When I stand before God at the end of my life,
I would hope that I would not have a
single bit of talent left, and could say,
'I used everything You gave me.'"*
~ Erma Bombeck

What did you want to be when you grew up? Or perhaps you are now grown up…and still deciding! I did not settle on elementary education until I was in my junior year of college. My career curiosities included: mathematician, businesswoman, physical therapist, nutritionist, nurse, communication's specialist, counselor, professional dancer, and more.

Eureka! One August afternoon in 1985, my path became straight. During a short nap, I had a dream from God. (I don't say this lightly.) In my dream I was sitting on a plaid, living room couch. In strolled Jesus. He walked towards me and pushed a snapshot directly in front of my face. I beheld children of various races and ages, smiling back at me. "What could this mean?" I quickly questioned. Jesus declared to me, "I have called you to be an educator."

Instantly I gazed at Jesus and responded like any anxious, career-seeking person would do. "Jesus, why did you wait so long to tell me?" What do you think He said? He said nothing.

Have you felt like God has occasionally been silent? Silence does not mean a lack of care on His part. On the contrary…He loves us…*all-knowingly*. Indeed, this inspiring race of life requires trust!

I awoke from that power nap feeling shocked back to life…as if jumper cables had been attached to the battery of my heart. God had called me to be an educator, and I was freshly inspired to earn two degrees in education.

The fit was amazing. Looking back on who God had created me to be, I had always thrived on learning and helping others learn as well. To illustrate, as a 14 year-old babysitter, I taught a six-year-old how to multiply. (Who wouldn't want a babysitter like that?) While on missions in the Appalachians, I used t-shirt slogans and pop cans to teach an illiterate teenager how to read. This young mountain man's eyes were instantly opened; I had a small part to play in that! How rewarding. How *inspiring*!

What inspiring aspects of life do you embrace? You can always ask God for your own jumper cable experience. Or He might just drop an idea into your heart. Either way, heed the call!

"The person born with a talent they are
meant to use will find their greatest
happiness in using it."
~ Johann Goethe

Date Your Mate

"*S*quish. Squish." How do you squeeze your toothpaste? Does it really matter? For the type A person, it does. The type B person could care less. Although I am a type A person in many respects, for some reason, I just let it all hang out with my toothpaste tactics. I gladly grab whatever kind of toothpaste is convenient (I don't care about the brand) and squirt a dot on my toothbrush (I don't care what kind, as long as it works.) A little dab will do me. On the other hand, my fine husband carefully squeezes his minty Crest toothpaste from the bottom up. Can you imagine the dexterity of our toothpaste tubes between my random squishes in the middle and Scott's vigilant foldings from the bottom? Each tube is a piece of artwork. To my husband's credit, he rolls with the punches very nicely, even when my turn with the tube makes it look like Mount St. Helen just erupted!

"The glowing magma emerges like red-hot
toothpaste from a long, wide crack
and then crawls into the Pacific,
creating a tall furious cloud of steam."
~ Robert Gross

After nearly 25 years of marriage, we have learned that the toothpaste dispensation is not a hill worth dying on! We laugh it off and seek to major on the majors in life instead of the minors. There is some truth to the old saying, "Don't make a mountain out of a molehill." Can you relate?

Sometimes the idiosyncrasies of our mates can bother us...or bless us! I choose to be blessed by my mate (at least that's my intention). How about you? Do you know what inspires me about Scott? First is his devotion to God. He loves God with all of his heart, soul, mind, and strength. Scott inspires me to be a better person. Even in private, Scott seeks to make wise choices and do what is right.

"Quality is never an accident; it is always the result of high intention, sincere effort, intelligent direction, and skillful execution; it represents the wise choice of many alternatives."
~ William Foster

Date your mate. That's what Scott (as a pastor) tells newly married couples. While raising children, this becomes increasingly more difficult for couples to do. For us, we must make a concerted effort to "schedule a date." Our dates consist of going for walks, out to eat, or perhaps to a movie. The most important element of the date, however, is giving the other person our undivided attention, thereby making sure our relationship is strongly connected. I appreciate the dating ground rules that Scott lays out for us:

1. No talking about the kids.
2. No talking about church (our calling and his profession).
3. No talking about Marathon Mission (the always fascinating non-profit I started).
4. No talking about money…well…sometimes!

So, what's left to talk about? At the beginning of our dinner dates I stare at my hubby for a few minutes and bite my tongue as my mind constantly reflects on the "taboo date topics." Then a wonderful, thought-inspiring, relational transformation occurs. We converse about magnificent memories. Before Scott's very eyes I begin to smile more and frown less. (Scott likes it when this serious momma smiles!)

"A smile is an inexpensive way
to change your looks."
~ Charles Gordy

I can't think of anything more inspiring in the marathon of life than holding my Honey's hand and dreaming about the future. Dreaming…(not the sleeping version!). When was the last time you allowed yourself that opportunity?

*"The future belongs to those who believe in
the beauty of their dreams."*
~ Eleanor Roosevelt

Marathon Mission is Born

What is a corporation? Frankly, at the turn of the 21st Century, words like profit, non-profit, and corporation seemed intimidating to me. I never took a lick of business or law classes. After all, I was just a pastor's wife, mom, teacher, and runner. What did I know about corporations? Back in 2003, not much! Yet today, I am the founder, president and CEO of Marathon Mission, a premier faith and community based non-profit umbrella corporation, comprised of compassionate, inspired walkers and runners.

"It is not the critic who counts...the credit belongs to the man who is actually in the arena...whose face is marred by dust and sweat and blood...who strives valiantly; who knows the great enthusiasm... the great devotion; who spends himself on a worthy cause...."
~ Theodore Roosevelt

Do you have a reason worth giving your time, talent, and resources to? My cause is Marathon Mission. Our story has been documented in numerous areas of media, including print, Internet, television, and radio. It's a contagious cause that continuously motivates participants, supporters, volunteers, and other charity heads.

It all began at the end of my "after childbearing" marathon with the Detroit Free Press/Flagstar Marathon in 2002. At the completion of those 26.2 miles, I realized that God supplied me with significant strength to finish that course, given my overall lapse of training for the past 17 years. While crossing the finish line, I was overcome with an attitude of gratitude and reasoned, "If people can do walk-a-thons, rock-a-thons, and bike-a-thons, why can't I do a marathon…for missions? I decided that in the following year I was going to actually train for and run the Detroit marathon again. Only next time, it would be for a reason beyond me! Have you found a means to distribute goodness to your sphere of influence, too?

"I resolved to stop accumulating and begin
the infinitely more serious and difficult task
of wise distribution."
~ Andrew Carnegie

Thus, I chose five missionary families that needed financial assistance: The Coates Family of Kenya; The Thompsons of Cleveland's Youth for Christ; the Keagys with Wycliffe Bible Translators in Peru; Joy of Jesus in Detroit; and "Heroes of the Faith" missionaries with First Assembly of God. How inspiring to utilize and coordinate my passions of running, people, service, and God…every day! I was to call my new found, humble marathon attempt, "Marathon Mission." Moreover, I expected it to be "one and done," meaning one Marathon Mission, and that would be it. Never did I expect what was to come.

"Is the rich world aware of how four billion of the six billion live? If we were aware, we would want to help out. We'd want to get involved."
~ Bill Gates

As the years have progressed, more and more walkers and runners of all ages and abilities have been inspired to use their strength for dozens of compassionate causes with Marathon Mission. (See www.marathonmission.net). Since Marathon Mission's conception, nearly 100 percent of the funds raised go directly to those worthy faith- and community-based works such as orphanages and food banks. This brings us back to those intimidating words: non-profit corporation. With free legal aid from Community Legal Resources and Wayne State University, Marathon Mission attained the much needed 501c3 legal status in 2006. As a result, donors may now also support Marathon Mission. This allows us to do what we do best, thereby enabling other faith- and community-based causes to keep running the race that is set before them. Marathon Mission inspires!

"Marathon Mission is not just a program.
It's a movement."
~ Scott A. Harper

Have you found a cause that puts a skip in your step? The greatest livers are the greatest givers!

STAGE 2

Preparation

"Do your very best to be found living
at your best."
(The Message)

Sharpening the Axe

"If I had six hours to chop down a tree,
I'd spend the first hour sharpening the axe."
~ Abraham Lincoln

Have you ever been thrust into a challenging situation for which you weren't prepared? Like a pop-quiz you needed to take or an impromptu speech you needed to make? To run an actual marathon of 26.2 miles, I understand that if I don't prepare well, I will not have the ability to finish. While too many training miles can actually cause a risk of injury, I also realize that there needs to be a foundation laid…a deposit of miles "in the bank" that I can carefully withdraw from, mile by mile, on marathon day.

Although there is a montage of individual approaches to marathon preparation, there is one component that every marathon runner has in common: *the long run.* (What do *you* like to do for the long run in life?) For the non-runner, a long run sounds like an accident waiting to happen…a major thorn in the side – or just plain crazy. Why would anyone willfully run 10-20 miles? Or perhaps, "What is wrong with someone who runs 10-20 miles?"

*"Hitting the ball was easy. Running around
the bases was the tough part."*
~ Mickey Mantle

I love my long runs. They simulate a marathon. However, I try to vary my running routes. When I first started my marathon running adventure, I continually ran the same path. Then, I discovered that I was being too narrow minded. So one day I turned the corner instead of going straight. Imagine that! I threw the control factor out the window, allowing myself to actually go down a street that I had never been before. How liberating!

Some days I'm in the "city" mood and will run on safe sidewalks along storefront streets with lots of traffic. The fumes aren't the greatest, but I do it because I just feel like being in the midst of the hustle and bustle. Other times I choose to journey through quiet neighborhoods or on an occasional dirt road (with a low "dog risk" factor!)

When was the last time you broke from your routine to allow yourself opportunity to experience new paths?

Sometimes I take water with me when I'm doing my long runs. There's definite wisdom to that. The trick is to drink before I'm thirsty, because by the time I feel thirsty, it's too late. I am already dehydrated!

*"Distant water won't quench
your immediate thirst."*
~ Chinese proverb

What do you enjoy doing on your Saturday mornings? While some Saturday long runs feel effortless, they actually require great will power and determination. They can even be a pain in the gluteus maximus! I'd rather be with my family, reading the paper, and eating the chocolate chip pancakes that my husband so kindly cooks for the kids. But pancakes are no substitute for miles! Fortunately, I've discovered that I can have my cake and eat it too. Or in my case, do my long run and eat those syrupy, Saturday pancakes with my name on them when I return.

If I did not do the long runs, I shutter to think of what would happen in the marathon. My legs would cramp sooner. My mind would play tricks on me. My heart and lungs would be running on overdrive. My shoulders would tighten, and my feet would want to fall off!

On the other hand, when I have prepared well with the long runs, then I am much more confident going into the marathon. Of course, there is always the fear of the unknown, but at least the lack of preparation will not be a factor in the success of that marathon for me! How can you prepare for tomorrow's opportunities?

"Unless a man has trained himself for his chance,
the chance will only make him look ridiculous."
~ J. B. Matthews

Miracle... Grow

There aren't many tasks in life that I run *away* from, but this one makes me shake in my boots: taking care of plants. This much I understand: there are indoor plants and outdoor plants. Years ago, I was given a very sentimental plant by Kathy Nutt that had been transported from our old, family cottage. Kathy has quite the knack and patience for nurturing plants to optimal health. I'm certain that she did not truly comprehend the risks involved in showering me with various forms of vegetation.

I knew the donated plant from Kathy needed sun, but what kind of sun? Direct? Indirect? Then there was the water factor. That's the one area where I really blew it. First, I would feel the soil to see if it was dry to the touch. If so, I would water it. Then my heart of mercy would overtake me, and I would think, *Was that enough water? Maybe it needs just a little bit more...poor thing!* Next, much to my bewilderment, and despite all of my watering attempts with tender loving care, the plant started to droop. *Poor thing. It must need MORE water,* I reasoned.

One would think that I would get it; I was drowning my wilting friend with the very thing that was supposed to help it.

"Never go to a doctor whose
office plants have died."
~ Erma Bombeck

Could too much of a good thing really not be a good thing?

Then there is the outdoor plant variety. As far as flowers go, I'm quite uninformed in terms of their botanical names and where such colorful dainties should be planted for optimum growth. When we first moved to our current home, I saw a perfect spot for my favorite, vibrant flowers…impatiens. (They are my favorite flowers by default. These were the only flowers I remember my family planting when I was a kid. Maybe it's genetic!) This "ideal" spot surrounded three, young maple trees evenly spaced on our front lawn near the road. With diligence I knelt down on my hands and knees to dig up the hard-packed soil full of roots. *These impatiens will look great right here,* I thought to myself. *But why are the neighbors laughing at me under their breath? Do they know something I don't?*

Apparently, yes. First, the location for the flowers was a terrible choice. Those impatiens got an awful beating with every ball that bounced by. If that wasn't enough, they were basking in far too much direct sunlight, which also caused them to wilt. There's that *wilt* word again.

"I'm just a wilting queen," I concluded. "I can't get it right with the plants inside or out!" So, what's a grown, ignorant gardener to do? For the inside variety, I have involuntarily donated all of my plants to heaven. Translation: we have no living plants in our house, except for the occasional flower-in-a-vase variety. However, I don't get too nervous over that kind, because vase flowers are going to die soon any way, so there's minimal risk involved ... a kind of no-fault insurance.

For the outside flowers, I still only plant impatiens, but now I plant them in the shade. I also learned the trick of applying a healthy dose of Miracle Grow... and praying for a miracle...that they will actually grow! Now, sometimes my merciful heart still overtakes me there, too, and I wonder, *Maybe they just need a little more Miracle Grow...poor things!*

Too much of a good thing is not a good thing. Sometimes we need to know when to say, "That's enough" – while the plants are still healthy and growing. What areas in life would you like to see flourish? How can you prepare more effectively to make that happen?

"He who never made a mistake
never made a discovery."
~ Samuel Smiles

39

A Cat, a Hat, and a Mouse

"The great of this world are those who
simply loved God more than others did."
~ A. W. Tozer

As a little girl, one of my favorite children's books
was *The Cat in the Hat* by Dr. Seuss. I liked the way
the words reasonably rhymed and made simple sense. I
also thought the Cat's hat looked funny.

What does your hat box look like? If you are like the
Harper family, you own several hats. In our closets we
have cowboy hats, stylish hats, snow hats, baseball caps,
furry hats, crocheted hats, thin hats, sports team hats,
and no-name hats. As a runner, sometimes I even wear
two hats to keep me warm in the winter.

I sport many symbolic hats in life too, such as the
hats of wife, mother, sister, daughter, aunt, friend,
neighbor, runner, Marathon Mission Director, educator, musician, chocolate lover, and pastor's wife. It's the
pastor's wife I'd like to focus on for a moment.

"You start out giving your hat,
then you give your coat, then your shirt,
then your skin and finally your soul."
~ Charles de Gaulle

What prepared me to be a pastor's wife of almost 25 years? First, both of my parents are true servants at heart. My father, Tom, is known among friends and strangers as being a generous man. My mother, Donna, used to tell me, "Honey, when you feel sad or lonely, go do something for someone else." Their example of providing for others a needed ride, meal, and even home instilled in me a desire to be a giver. My family viewed meeting a God-directed need as a privilege. I do, too. This mindset is critical in being an effective pastor's wife.

Some pastor's wives labor to put on that hat. For me, I take no credit; I believe that I was just born with that hat on. As a high school freshman I enjoyed the rewards of counseling at the inner-city camp called Joy of Jesus. Unbeknownst to me, my future husband was doing the same thing. As suburban teens we would drive ourselves into Detroit to lend a hand up and not just a hand out. That was the motto of Joy of Jesus.

Moreover, as a senior in high school, I would drive one hour each Saturday afternoon to a county detention facility for juveniles my own age. Why did I do this? My heart longed for the teens to be set free from their chains of inner turmoil. I knew that God was the only one who could give them that peace that passes all understanding.

My college years at Oral Roberts University also prepared me to be a pastor's wife. Serving others through Christian service councils and student missions programs fit me perfectly. Then, marrying Scott Harper was like frosting on the cake. Fortunately, we are both called to pastoral ministry, and God gives us the grace to do it.

I can't change the oil in the car or sew worth beans, but I can choose to flow in the gifts that God created me to give. God prepared me to do this, even though I did not know it at the time. The shoe fits…and I humbly wear it!

What's in your hand to do? How has God prepared you for what you are doing now? Take a look in the mirror. You have been born with many hats, but what good is a hat if it's not on your head? Make sure the God-ordained hats stay on your head…not in your hand.

> *"If you can dream it, you can do it.*
> *Always remember that this whole thing*
> *was started with a dream and a mouse."*
> ~ Walt Disney

Sweet Tooth Trouble

"There's always free cheese in the mouse traps,
but the mice there ain't happy."

~ Anonymous

*I*ve always had a major sweet tooth, particularly as a child. When I was five years old I privately ate 10 hand-sized cream cakes! Imagine that! My stomach took years to recover. Unfortunately, one would think I would learn my lesson, but my desire for other forms of sweets, like Reese's Peanut Butter Cups, just grew exponentially with every passing year. By the time I was eight or nine, I had a serious problem.

What tempted you as a child? The temptation that lay before me was too much for me to bear. One of my older teenage brothers, Mark, had a thriving lawn business. He would frequently empty his pockets after a hard-working day and put the change on his nightstand. (Just the right height for my eyes to gaze directly at all of that money!) I quickly realized that if I carefully took a few strategic, large, silver coins from his collection, he might never know. You see, he was a diligent worker who kept bringing in the dough...*to me*! "We're in the money!" I started to sing to myself.

It wasn't really the money that I wanted – It was the candy that I could buy with the money! Unfortunately,

43

I wanted the sweet treats but was not willing to work for them myself. Mark was splendid at earning the money, and I was a sneaky pro at stealing it.

With my pockets weighed down by the coins (not the brown ones, but the robust, silver ones), I walked at least one-half mile with my childhood friend, Holly, to the Chippewa Party Store. Every time I flittered into that place, I felt like I entered heaven. So many choices…so many chocolates! (No wonder I liked the movie, *Willy Wonka and the Chocolate Factory*!) I came from the Nutt family with five kids, where I was the youngest and had to jockey to get remaining morsels of after-dinner desserts. I was desperate for the smooth taste, the creamy feeling of a melting piece of chocolate to caress my watering mouth.

"There are four basic food groups:
milk chocolate, dark chocolate,
white chocolate, and chocolate truffles."
~ Anonymous

This "peek, sneak, steal, walk, buy, and eat" candy process lasted several months. Then I went to the dentist. Oops. My party was over! I had eight cavities. Yes, eight. I couldn't believe it! What happened? It could very well have been that I did not brush my teeth enough. (Who could possibly keep up with all of that candy collected in my mouth?) However, the issue was deeper. I knew in my heart that stealing from my brother was wrong. The guilt I felt was so heavy, my heart felt like it was being crushed. I also knew that I had been lazy. If I wanted to buy some candy, I should have been inventive enough to find an honest way to earn the money. I wanted to eat candy and be merry, with no sacrifice, no hard work, and no preparation on my part.

"Laziness may appear attractive,
but work gives satisfaction."
~ Anne Frank

I learned my lesson well. First, I confessed my mistakes to my understanding brother. He was amazed at the masterminding skills I possessed and actually laughed when he learned that I received eight cavities for my foolishness! Next, my appetite for candy was drastically curtailed. I remember thinking, *Lisa, you've got to change!* At that ripe, young age I had to gather myself up by my bootstraps and start to work for what I wanted. As for the cream cakes, that's all she wrote!

How are you working for what you want? Today, will you take one small step in that direction?

"Success is not final, failure is not fatal:
it is the courage to continue that counts."
~ Winston Churchill

Make Your Omelet Now

"Do not wait; the time will never be
'just right'. Start where you stand,
and work with whatever tools you may have
at your command, and better tools will
be found as you go along."
~ Napoleon Hill

*W*hen I was a student at Oral Roberts University, Ron Luce (Teen Mania/Battle Cry founder) asked me, "Lisa, what one thing would you do if you knew you couldn't fail?" That powerful question has been engrained in me ever since then. As a pastor's wife since my ORU days, I have loved asking others that question. At first they pause. They have to think for a moment. All of us are so used to putting limitations on ourselves. We rarely dare to dream beyond tomorrow (or even today), because we don't want to risk failure, particularly in the eyes of others.

"You can't make an omelet
without breaking eggs."
~ Proverb

Have you ever considered the notion that you could actually do the impossible? Today I dare to dream by asking this question of myself: What one thing would I do if I knew I could not fail? I would become a published author by writing this book. I have never written a complete book before, however, I have been fortunate to write a chapter as a co-author in a few books, such as *Your Exceptional Life Begins Now* (Aloha Publishing) and *From Fairbanks to Boston, 50 Great U.S. Marathons* (Rainmaker Publishing).

What intimidates you? The authoring process can be an intimidating one for me, but I'm ready to put in the miles and persevere. Looking back on my life, I can also see how some of my "base mileage" as a ready writer has prepared me well for this new venture.

As a child I loved to write heart-warming, honest letters, particularly to my folks in Chicago. During my teenage years I painted rocks for my family, friends, and teachers, thereafter putting their names, the meanings of their names, and creative phrases on each rock. As a college student I journaled often and loved to express my feelings through the written word. As a youth pastor's wife, one Christmas I wrote over 30 personal poems for each of our Powerhouse youth leaders at our beloved St. Clair Shores Assembly of God (The Shores Church) in Michigan. Then, as a mother, I penned painful letters to each of my five children who were not born alive due to miscarriages. I also like to write encouraging Bible studies. Most recently, I have found myself writing persuasive letters of recommendation for exceptional young men and women who are applying to various universities.

So why do I write this book *now*? I write now because I feel compelled to make a legacy while I'm still alive. Legacies can start while you're living, not just after you've kicked the bucket! Sure, I have plenty of insecurities. I don't know about building a marketing plan, designing the cover, obtaining registrations, interior book designs, and taking the book to print. I could certainly allow these unknowns to paralyze me like a deer staring into headlights, or I can say, "I don't know, but I'm determined to find out!" God has been preparing me for this specific time. By His grace and through unassuming perseverance, I am becoming a published author!

God has been preparing you all of your life for such a time as this, too. Now what are you waiting for? What would *you* do if you knew you could not fail? How can you turn your intimidations into triumphs?

STAGE 3

Perspiration

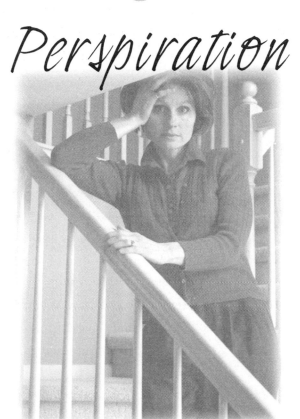

*"Anyone who meets a testing challenge head-on
and manages to stick it out is mighty fortunate.
For such persons loyally in love with God,
the reward is life and more life."*

(The Message)

You're Glowing

"Success is 10 percent inspiration
and 90 percent perspiration."
~ Thomas Alva Edison

"You're glowing!" That's how my childhood gymnastics instructor, Frances Borgo, referred to perspiration. Less sophisticated people might just call it sweat. Whatever you want to call it, God made our bodies to perspire, and it can actually be good for us.

Perspiration occurs when our sweat glands secret a fluid (made up primarily of water and salt) through the pores of our skin. Frankly, perspiration acts as our bodies' temperature gauge.

How do you feel when you get too hot? When you exercise, your body begins to heat up. When I first began to run in college, my generous Uncle Tim and Aunt Marlene gave me a well-meaning Christmas gift: a double-layered, all-cotton, bright red, hooded sweatshirt. I was so excited to have something warm to run in while in Michigan! Yet, my ignorance got the best of me; as I ran outside in the wintertime in my romping red sweatshirt, that covering got wetter and heavier by the minute. As the years went on, I realized that I should be running in layers made of lighter, moisture-wicking fabric when possible, not thick cotton. Folks, there's a reason why cloth diapers are made of cotton…it's for absorption! Not wanting to feel like I was wearing a wet diaper, I gradually switched over to clothing that allowed my body to sweat and allowed those fluids to evaporate.

As a runner, I also perspire when the weather is hot and humid. During some of my college days in Tulsa, Oklahoma, I would run two times a day, 60 miles a week…running in the afternoon in 100-plus degree weather. Ahhh, nothing like a hot breeze blowing right into your nostrils! We would perspire just by walking to class, not to mention running along the banks of the Arkansas River. I quickly learned that to perspire less, I should run more in the morning, before the blazing hot sun dominated the sky.

"Patience, persistence, and perspiration make
an unbeatable combination for success."
~ Napolean Hill

Another factor in my "runner's glow" is how fast I run. Usually at the beginning of my Michigan Marathons, I'm rather chilly. Yet it doesn't take long before I start shedding the layers of clothing as my body heats up. By the end of the 26.2 miles, I'm plenty warm and drenched with perspiration, with salt (dried sweat) on my forehead to prove it.

With marathon training, I do easy-paced, distance running. However, if I need to quickly get warm, I sprint to the next streetlight. The oven inside me just heats up like a bowl of hot tamales. Humorously, there is no way that I can maintain that sprinting pace for any length of time (unlike my good husband, Scott, who used to run 4-minute miles!), but it sure does stoke up my core temperature!

"Success seems to be connected to action.
Successful people keep moving."
~ Conrad Hilton

Some people just hate to perspire, bless their hearts. Their pores are missing out on a good cleansing. According to Ezinearticles.com, "The shifting of hot-cold gets the circulation flowing and flushes the body from the inside out and outside in."

Next time you are embarrassed or upset about perspiring, think twice. Don't let it stop you. Most good things in life don't come by sitting on the couch. Go ahead and exercise outside when you can. Breathe deeply. Dress properly. Pick the best time of the day. Be set free - and get yourself a strong deodorant!

"Do you know why conductors live so long?
Because we perspire so much."
~ John Barbirolli

The Techy Tangle

"Technology is like a fish. The longer it stays on the shelf, the less desirable it becomes."
~ Andrew Heller

Some people are right brained. Others are left. A few have no brain. No, just kidding! Yet, I often feel like my brain is in left field when it comes to technological advances.

Take the computer, for example. Who came up with such weird terminology? *Mouse?* I don't want a mouse in my house! *Cursor?* No, sir, we don't curse in our home either. *Tower?* Sure. Take me to it. I've always wanted to visit the Eiffel Tower. *Ram?* Is that like a buffalo with horns on it? *Web?* Do you mean *Charlotte's Web?* Oh, I love that childhood story. Or do you mean spider web? Well, there are plenty of those behind my computer, too.

How many times have your computers needed resuscitation? I know I have lost count. Recently, it would have cost us at least $600 for a traveling computer geek to come to our house and fix all of our computer problems. That's just for the "extended stay" home service call – the guy might as well stay for dinner!

"The most overlooked advantage
of owning a computer is that if they foul up,
there's no law against whacking them around a bit."
~ Eric Porterfield

Our most recent crisis occurred when the monitor of our flat-screened Dell E310 went completely black. What? Black? I need to see some lights or at least a moving blue bar along the screen somewhere! I was faced with a dilemma that many of you have considered, but few of you may admit to. Should I just chuck the whole thing in the garbage? No, it's too costly. Thus, instead of thrusting it, I laid my hands on the rebellious box and prayed something like this:

"Oh God of heaven and earth. Nothing is hidden from you. You said, 'Let there be light,' and there was. God, if you parted the Red Sea and helped Peter walk on the water, you can certainly speak life into this rotten computer and bring light to my darkness. Do it now, Lord! Revival fire, fall on my computer! Restore and refresh it by your Spirit!"

Sometimes we are called to be a part of the solution to our prayers, so I thought I would help God out by calling for technical support. (That takes the patience of Job.) With reluctant forbearance, I dialed the 1-800 number, only to get various non-human prompts on the other end. Suddenly I found myself screaming the requested responses like a fanatic. My answers to the impersonal questions went something like this: "TECHNICAL SUPPORT! DESKTOP! YES! NO! I DON'T KNOW! YOU TELL ME!"

Once I did get a live person on the other end, it was obvious to me that the professional was located somewhere else in the world. Now I am all for international relations and world peace, but when I need a translator to understand my own technical supporter, I exclaimed, "May day! May day!"

Next, my on-call helper asked me to disconnect and reconnect several plugs from the back of the select boxes. No, Lord. God help me. Not the plugs! That's where the webs are, and the mouse and tower are not far from it. Why doesn't someone color code those tangled plugs? That's where the real web begins right there!

Without a little perspiration, I hear that nothing good comes, so I'll persevere. Sometimes we need to follow instructions even if we don't truly understand – God often prefers it that way.

"They have computers, and they have other weapons of mass destruction."
~ Janet Reno

How can you turn your frustrations, that often lead to perspirations, into achievements?

The Summer Within

"I am indebted to my father for living,
but to my teacher for living well."
~ Alexander the Great

*W*hich teacher do you remember the most? My high school English teacher at Southfield Christian School, David Cochrane, was the hardest teacher I ever had, including college and graduate professors. I had heard about the 20-page, final exam from my older, and salutatorian brother, Jeffrey Nutt. Some students pretended to lift weights with the exam when it landed on their desks.

Such a lengthy exam should be illegal, my sophomore (meaning "wise fool") mind reasoned. How could I possibly prepare for that? Nouns, verbs, pronouns, adjectives, adverbs, prepositions, conjunctions, interjections...I diligently studied to keep them all straight. Do you remember their functions today? Then there were his expectations of our three-point essays, including details, examples, and a well-developed thesis statement.

Mr. Cochrane also had an eccentric personality, which some students mocked. I didn't dare ask it aloud, but why did he glide across the room with his duck-like feet out-turned, seemingly bouncing on the balls of his feet? With all of Mr. Cochrane's mannerisms, including the way he held his chalk and the super-human demands, I liked the guy. He became one of my favorite teachers because he challenged me, and I trusted his college-preparatory judgment.

Have you ever had a dream that seemed to randomly reoccur from time to time? Mine always has to do with school. In the dream I'm either surprised by a test, forgetful of my locker combination, or not allowed to graduate from college because the academic advisors "discovered" on graduation day that I was one class too short! I think that the stress I experienced from Mr. Cochrane's class still has something to do with this reoccurring dream. Can anyone say, "All-nighter"?

"The task of the excellent teacher is to stimulate 'apparently ordinary' people to unusual effort."
~ K. Patricia Cross

I was privileged to have Mr. Cochrane as my instructor for two more classes my senior year: College Writing and World Literature. For College Writing, I was sufficiently intimidated in learning the college study skills that I actually read and recorded my notes on tape, listening to them while I took a shower the morning of the test. I was scared silly.

"Courage is being scared to death,
but saddling up anyway."
~ John Wayne

In World Literature, Mr. Cochrane required students to do a variety of projects, along with our pressure-packed papers. I'm grateful to him for this because I went out of my comfort zone. To illustrate the *Brother's Karamazov*, I did an interpretive dance. To expound upon *A Canticle for Lebowitz*, I attempted my first legitimate still drawing of a pair of well-worn sandals, which hangs on my wall today. For another piece of literature, I played a classical piano selection that reflected the mood of the writer.

"In the midst of winter, I found there was
within me an invincible summer."
~ Albert Careb

If it weren't for Mr. Cochrane, I never would have stretched on my own to do art, music and dance like that. Love believes the best in others; Mr. Cochrane believed the best in me. I went on to become valedictorian of my senior class. I did not have the highest IQ in the class. I just perspired, studied, and persevered to become the best student that I could be. Mr. Cochrane took an apparently ordinary student and made me a winner.

Who's your Mr. Cochrane? In turn, who can you teach to saddle up and ride?

"A teacher affects eternity;
he can never tell where his influence stops."
~ Henry Adams

Amazing Grace

"Life is either a daring adventure or nothing."
~ Helen Keller

*H*ave you ever had someone sneak up on you? "Pitter, patter, clip, clop." I could hear the fast footsteps behind me as I crossed Nevada Avenue on my way into Bethesda Missionary Temple that dark, April, Wednesday night. As a 17-year-old suburban gymnast who also loved my city church, I had just driven 20 miles to get there.

By the time I had arrived at this mega church by 1980s standards, the parking was scarce, so I had to park across a busy street and down a few blocks. When I arrived, I was just finishing listening to *Amazing Grace* on the radio. It was odd for me to hear that song over the airwaves, so I parked and waited until it was done. Then I got out of my grandpa's old, silver, Mercury Marquis and briskly started walking toward the main church entrance.

"Pitter, patter, clip, clop." What was that noise? I immediately turned around to see a man, dressed in camouflage pants and red tennis shoes, pointing a gun right at my face.

"Ma'am. Would you get back in your car please?" He rather politely asked.

What might go through your mind in that split second, if you were me? I quickly rationalized, *If I comply, then I'll have to do what he tells me. Who knows what he would make me do?* So, with all of the adolescent courage I could muster, I firmly told the gunman, "No, I *won't!*" (They don't call me Hurricane Lisa for nothing!)

With that, I ran as fast as I could in my heels and skirt through the parking lot and over Nevada Avenue. Half in shock and half infused with adrenaline, I continued that street journey that seemed to last forever. (I guess this makes me a runner in high school after all!) *This is like a movie!* I really thought. *Am I going to get shot in the back? I wonder if I'll make it to the main door alive.*

Finally, I thrust my body into the House of God, my true refuge in more ways than one! What a relief: I had made it to the foyer without a bullet in my back. Ushers came over to "greet" me. (Wasn't that nice?). I told them about the gunman and how thankful I was that the gun wasn't loaded (otherwise, I figured, the gunman would have shot me.) While I was describing the crime, another woman rushed into the lobby and yelled, "This guy just stole my car!"

"The best armor is staying out of gun-shot."
~ Italian proverb

Indeed, that criminal took her car, with her in it! Soon she escaped. The gunman continued driving. A church security patrol car followed the gunman as he drove like a maniac over curbs and into signs. Next, the gunman exited the car, walked up to the security man, pointed his gun at his window, and shot!

Fortunately, no one was hurt. The authorities captured the convict and confiscated his gun (a sawed-off shot gun). Hurricane Lisa had been through the ringer. After being taken by police to an inner-city precinct to identify the man, I was kindly driven back to my abandoned car in the desolate parking lot that midnight. It was a long, lonely drive home, but can you guess what song I heard again on the radio to keep me company?

"Amazing grace, how sweet the sound,
that saved a wretch like me..."

In your marathon of life, which moments caused you to perspire the most? How did God show you His amazing grace through each one?

Sleep Deprived

*D*o you have a favorite cop movie? Picture the thrill of watching it. Then let your imagination join with me in this true, nail-biting, heart-racing, sweat-producing Harper escapade.

> *"All battles are fought by scared men*
> *who'd rather be some place else."*
> ~ John Wayne

Sleep has continually been a vital commodity for the Harpers. Once, while visiting my parents (Tom and Kathy Nutt) in suburban Chicago, our youngest daughter Jasmine woke up in the middle of the night, confused by a dream and unsure of her surroundings. She began to scream uncontrollably. With seven sleeping people in a compact townhouse, I unsuccessfully tried my level best to quiet her.

What would you do then? I quickly scooped up the noisy, flailing Jasmine and promptly proceeded outside. When we stepped out the front door which was just below the neighbor's bedroom window, Jasmine yelled like a wild child, "No! No! NO!" Doing what any quick-thinking mother would do, I put my hand over her mouth, which I'm sure appeared as if I were trying to suffocate or kidnap my own child.

I called upon all of my speed work in running (not really, if you recall, because I am a slower, long distance runner), opened the side door to our family-friendly, Econoline van, and thrust my daughter in there as fast as you could shake a stick.

"When you are a mother, you are never really alone in your thoughts. A mother always has to think twice, once for herself and once for her child."
~ Sophia Loren

"Mommy, what are you doing?" Jasmine asked. By this time her outbursts had stopped and I was looking like the one who was out of control! I proceeded to explain to Jasmine the importance of being quiet in the house while people are sleeping. Then I heard a police car slowly approaching. What a movie! Chicago's finest started shining spotlights on the front of the townhouses, searching for a criminal. *I can't believe this!* I pondered. I felt like Maria Von Trapp, hiding in the cemetery with her youngest daughter Gretl, in that famous film, *The Sound of Music.*

To avoid any spotlight induced shadows, we slid down to the floor of our van. When the police car circled around the block, I quickly pulled down the shades. Jasmine was clueless. I'm sure I appeared like an out of control mother.

Should I step out of the van, as if it's a hold up, and

explain the sleep deprivation dilemma to the officer? Would he really understand, or would I be taken away forever from my four beloved children?

Wait. There's more. If that wasn't enough, a helicopter decided to fly overhead. I even heard them say something from a speaker while shining their lights down on the rooftops. Were they telling me to come out with my hands up? *But what have I done wrong?* I asked. *I was just trying to help everyone sleep.*

The call to flight kicked in. I decided to take the now-silent and bemused Jasmine into my arms one more time. Lickety-split, we synchronized our dash back *into* the townhouse when the spotlights were elsewhere.

Once inside, I ducked, for fear that they might shine the lights into the townhouse windows. By this time, Jasmine had forgotten why she woke up in the first place. After I put her back to bed, I couldn't resist crawling to the window and peeking through the blinds to see if there was more drama to come. Talk about perspiration!

> *"The hand that rocks the cradle usually is attached to someone who isn't getting enough sleep."*
> ~ John Fiebig

Is there currently an area in your life that's making you perspire? What are some healthy ways to manage your stress levels and actually flourish in the midst of the challenge?

STAGE 4

Initiation

*"There has never been the slightest doubt
in my mind that the God who started this
great work in you would keep at it
and bring it to a flourishing finish."*

(The Message)

Flipping the Switch

"Most people run a race to see who is fastest.
I run a race to see who has the most guts."
~ Steve Prefontaine

Who is the most courageous person you know? The gutsiest runner I know is my wonderful husband and coach, Scott Andrew Harper. Scott ran cross-country, indoor track, and outdoor track for 11 consecutive years. In fact, Scott has run over 330 races! At his running career pinnacle, Scott was a NCAA Division I All-American and eighth in the nation in the two-mile run (8:38).

With Scott's wealth of racing experience, I asked him about his fastest high school race, particularly the start, the initiation.

Scott's most successful high school meet was the Southern Michigan Association league meet in Michigan his senior year. He won the mile in a blistering time of 4:14! Scott attributes the success of that race to a few factors. First, being relaxed and playful before the race helped. He grabbed the opponent's mascot teddy bear and ran around with it! (This would be the total opposite of yours truly, by the way.) Staying relaxed *before* the race helped Scott achieve maximum results.

However, once the gun went off, Scott became like

a horse racing for the barn. In his words, he "flipped the switch," and said to himself, "Okay. It's time to GO!"

Go he did. Scott had talked with God before the race, and unlike any other race before or since, God spoke to his heart and told him precisely what his split times would be: 60 seconds, 2:05, 3:12, and 4:14. That is exactly what happened. For the first 220 yards Scott positioned himself in front, ready to cut in when permissible. He did not want to get boxed in or allow another runner to impede his stride. Running in front, foot loose and fancy free, Scott broke the tape as the winner.

> *"I believe God made me for a purpose,*
> *but He also made me fast."*
> ~ Eric Liddell

Did Scott always break the tape first? No, Scott will be the first to tell you that he did not win all of his races. Some disappointing races still haunted him, but by focusing on the next race, he was able to persevere with anticipation.

Of all the exceptional runners of antiquity, our favorite is the Olympian-turned-missionary, Eric Liddell. The Oscar-winning movie, *Chariots of Fire*, depicts Liddell's famous post-race address to a rain-soaked crowd:

> *You came to see a race today. To see someone win.*
> *It happened to be me. But I want you to do more*

than just watch a race. I want you to take part in it. I want to compare faith to running in a race. It's hard. It requires concentration of will, energy of soul. You experience elation when the winner breaks the tape – especially if you've got a bet on it. But how long does that last? You go home. Maybe your dinner's burnt. Maybe you haven't got a job. So who am I to say, "Believe, have faith," in the face of life's realities? I would like to give you something more permanent, but I can only point the way. I have no formula for winning the race. Everyone runs in her own way, or his own way. And where does the power come from, to see the race to its end? From within. Jesus said, 'Behold, the Kingdom of God is within you. If with all your hearts, you truly seek Me, you shall ever surely find Me.' If you commit yourself to the love of Christ, then that is how you run a straight race.
~ Eric Liddell

What strategies can you implement into your race of life that will help you to start strong and have faith in your daily journeys?

The Little Box

"Grow old along with me. The best is yet to be."
~ Robert Browning

*H*ow did you meet your mate? Not many people meet their mates when they are 15 years old, but I did. This initiation into my race of a lifetime with Scott Harper actually happened at a Joy of Jesus camp staff meeting. I was a freshman in high school and Scott was a senior. I remember pondering, *Oh, he's really nice, but he probably thinks I'm too young.* Scott thought, *Hey, she's really nice, but she's too young.*

Four years later and one thousand miles from home, we met again at college in Tulsa, Oklahoma. (We both grew up in Michigan, only six miles apart.) Once again, Scott was a senior and I was a freshman. What goes around comes around! God has a plan, and time has a way of changing things.

"Life is all about timing…the unreachable becomes reachable, the unavailable become available, the unattainable…attainable. Have the patience. Wait it out. It's all about timing."
~ Stacey Charter

While our courtship began on our college campus, the last half of it was long distance. I wanted to love the one I was with, but I wasn't with the one I loved! Has this ever happened to you? Scott returned to Michigan to start pastoral ministry. I was finishing my elementary degree back in Oklahoma.

Then came December 19, 1985. I was home in Michigan on winter break. Christmas music was in the air, and mistletoes were everywhere! Do you know what that means?

Scott planned a special evening for us. First, with roses in hand, he picked me up in a *washed,* red, Ford Escort. Dressed in a dapper, tan, woolen suit coat, matching plaid scarf, and a suit right out of *GQ Magazine,* Scott looked smashing.

We headed towards a lovely Japanese riverside restaurant, where we had our own room and sat low to the ground. There, Scott took off his snazzy, leather shoes.

Something sure seems fishy, I reasoned. *If Scott was ever going to propose to me, THIS would be the night.* We proceeded to exchange Christmas gifts. My carefully wrapped Christmas boxes for Scott consisted of running shoes (of course) and warm winter gloves. Scott had two gifts for me, too, but where was "the little box?"

Like any honest maiden in love, I wanted what was in that box, and I wanted Scott to pop the question. Scott opened his presents with gratitude. Then, my man had the gall to comment, "Lisa, I hope you weren't getting your expectations up for tonight." Wittily I responded, "Scott, my expectations are in God!"

Was he playing mind games with me? Of course my expectations were sky high. I mean, the washed car, the scarlet roses, the snazzy attire, the intimate restaurant – the works! This night *seemed* like the initiation of a new life together. Starting line running tips flashed before me: Stay composed. Don't get boxed in. Position yourself to reach your goals (like being engaged by Christmas)!

It was my turn to open my two gifts, with no little box in sight. First, Scott gave me a paperback book about evangelism. Great. Just what I always wanted! My face portrayed the most insincere smile this side of the Mississippi.

Next, I held a wooden plaque up to my hopeful eyes and read this inscription on the golden template: "Lisa, will you marry me?" Out came the little box, too. I met my running partner for life. What a proposal. What an initiation!

My heart to you is given:
Oh, do give yours to me;
We'll lock them up together,
and throw away the key.
~ Frederick Saunders

What goodness can you initiate and impart into the life of someone else today?

Rise and Shine

"Eat a live toad the first thing in the morning,
and nothing worse will happen to you
the rest of the day."
~ Unknown

*A*re you a morning person or an evening person?
Being a mother who had four children in seven
years, I had to become "all things to all men." Mornings
were never more challenging for me than when my son,
Jonathan, was a young toddler.

As a bubbly, smiling young fellow, Jonathan was
either exceedingly happy, or terribly sad. For some reason
his internal clock was confused as to what truly con-
stituted morning and what defined evening.

When Jonathan was strong enough to climb out of
his crib (not long after he turned one), he did just that.
His motor skills were so far ahead of his brain that there
was absolutely no way to reason with him. So, after he
continually escaped from his wooden crib in our Davisburg, Michigan, home, Scott and I decided to take the
crib out of his room and put a mattress on the floor.
Unfortunately, Jonathan didn't even understand that he
was supposed to sleep on the mattress, so he slept for
several weeks, Winnie the Pooh blanket and all, right on
his carpeted floor near the door.

"I'd like mornings better if they started later."

~ Unknown

For Jonathan, it didn't matter what time the clock said...4 AM...5 AM...If he was awake, then it was time to start his day. True, Jonathan was a lovable little lad, but I became exhausted as he continually walked out into the hallway to start *his* day in what seemed like the middle of *my* night. (How do you feel when you are burning the candle at both ends?)

Once, I gently guided Jonathan back into his room and over to the double-paned window. Pulling the narrow blinds apart just a bit, the two of us peeked through the window. (He liked that, but I really wasn't in the mood for peek-a-boo!)

Can you guess what I whispered to him with sleepy sincerity? "Jonathan, dear. Do you see that glowing thing up in the sky? That is the moon. That is not the sun! The moon is for night time; the sun is for day." Although my intentions were noble, my motherly explanation fell on deaf ears. Jonathan kept waking up before the cock even crowed.

"If people were meant to pop out of bed,
we'd all sleep in toasters."

~ Unknown

I have heard that old saying, "If you can't beat 'em, join 'em," so I did. Every morning during this delicate phase of Jonathan's life I would quietly take him downstairs to our library of books. I placed his cute, pajama-clad, rolly polly body on the carpet, right next to the shelf where the books were easily within his reach.

"One morning I shot an elephant in my pajamas.
How he got into my pajamas, I'll never know."
~ Groucho Marx

Many times I could barely keep my eyelids opened, so I resorted to the best babysitter in the world: books! Jonathan would pull his Barney books from the shelves, at which time I surrounded his cross-legged frame with them. Books in front, books on his knees, books at his back, books where we pleased. Little did I know that this exposure to books would instill in Jonathan a love for reading that thrives to this day. I wouldn't trade those sleepless nights for anything.

Sometimes our days don't begin like we want them to. I've learned to laugh more, go with the flow, and take a dose of morning medicine from Billy Graham:

"I can tell you that God is alive,
because I talked to Him this morning."
~ Billy Graham

How can you make your mornings bright? Will you join me in choosing to get up on "the right side of the bed?"

Good-byes and Hellos

According to wordnet.princeton.edu/perl/webwn, "initiation" is defined as, "The act of starting something for the first time; introducing something new."

What was it like for you to start a new job? Embarking on a new job is an intense initiation these days. Factors such as a finicky economy or a faultering family situation often require occupational changes and moves. Some fluctuating seasons of employment are our choice; others are thrust upon us without warning.

"For many people a job is more than an income –
it's an important part of who we are. So a career
transition of any sort is one of the most unsettling
experiences you can face in your life."
~ Paul Clitheroe

As a pastor's family, we have served in several Michigan churches. Each time the arrival at the new was usually easier than the departure from the old, for we grew to love each group immensely. Fortunately, after every good-bye there is another hello.

Our journey started when Scott was a circuit rider type of preacher at the age of 23. Not only was he the youth pastor at Davisburg Methodist (where we were married), but at the same time he served as the senior pastor at Mt. Bethel, a 150- year-old congregation in the country. What a rich history! That congregation loved the young blood that we brought.

"Though no one can go back and make a brand new start, anyone can start from now and make a brand new ending."
~ Unknown

Our travels then took us to The Shores Church (St. Clair Shores Assembly of God) where the Powerhouse youth leaders and youth groups were top-notch. When things are going well at your place of employment, do you really want to leave? No, and neither did we, but our Sr. Pastor Paul Sundell was retiring (deservedly so). It was time to move.

What's the largest step of faith you've ever taken? Scott and I took a sizeable step of faith to move from a congregation of 700 to a congregation of 7. (Yes, that's a difference of two zeros!) So it was, and all seven of them left. God had a plan for our family and Hope Alive church in Holly. The church steadily grew, and we sensed God's timing for a new initiative.

"Why can't we get all the people together in the world that we really like and then just stay together? I guess that wouldn't work. Someone would leave.

Someone always leaves. Then we would have to say
good-bye. I hate good-byes. I know what I need.
I need more hellos."
~ Charles M. Schulz

Our next "hello" was at First Assembly of God in Dearborn Heights, Michigan. Scott served 10 rewarding years as their senior pastor. The church wrapped their gracious arms around us and helped to raise our four children. Genuine love overflowed from First Assembly, for which we will always be grateful.

"Some people come into our lives and quickly go.
Some stay for a while, leave footprints on our
hearts, and we are never, ever the same."
~ Flavia Weedn

Connection Church in Canton, MI would be our next destination. Pastor Rocky and the congregation excelled at connecting people to God.

Thereafter, Clare Assembly of God in Clare, MI welcomed us with genuine kindness. What a privilege to serve this fine congregation for many years. The best is yet to come!

How many jobs have you actually relished? We have enjoyed every place that we have served. Such is not the case for the typical employee. Whatever your current lot in life, if it's time to embrace the new, then step out boldly. Express appreciation. Show your team spirit. Find a mentor. Work diligently.

> *"He who has begun a good work in you*
> *will carry it on to completion."*
> ~ Philippians 1:6 (NIV)

How can you demonstrate initiation as a self-starter? What are some benefits that you expect to reap from all of the good that you purposely sow?

Patchwork Quilt

"Strangers are friends you have yet to meet."
~ Anonymous

How do you feel about meeting strangers? How do you feel when they come into your home? *Strangers.* For most of us, that word brings a negative connotation and sends chills down our spines! We are told to avoid strangers at all costs, go the other way; don't look them in the eye. We must be wise and careful, but I'd like to respectfully challenge the mindset that all strangers are dangerous and untrustworthy. After all, if *I* were to meet *you* for the first time, you would initially be a stranger to me, but I dare say that you would not be dangerous or alarming – at least not most of you.

Because of fear, intimidation, and insecurity, too many of us miss the boat in meeting wonderful strangers who turn into remarkable friends. True, we must incorporate careful discernment, but being overly skeptical of strangers is narrow-minded and limiting. Don't throw out the baby with the bath water, and don't assume every stranger is a bad person.

Thanksgiving at the Harper House has provided unique opportunities for us to practice what we preach. Our friendship initiative occurs with international students from Eastern Michigan University and Chi Alpha.

Some of these students don't have a home in which to celebrate the meaningful Thanksgiving holiday.

When we first became aware of the need, Scott and I had a choice to make. We could have said, "No, we don't want to have them interrupt our own family traditions. We don't understand their ways, and they don't understand ours. Plus, more guests means we might have to cook two turkeys!"

"Internationalism does not mean
the end of individual nations.
Orchestras don't mean the end of violins."
~ Golda Meir

Instead we enthusiastically opened our home. "We'd love to share with you our traditions of giving thanks to God with a grateful heart. Please share with us your traditions and cultures, and bring a native dish to pass!"

That was one of the best family decisions we've ever made! Our children and other relatives have now had the world come to them. In fact, our international guests have come from Thailand, Taiwan, Japan, Korea, the Caribbean, Vietnam, Brazil, Mexico, Spain, Germany, Egypt, Palestine, Kuwait, Iran, Nigeria, Israel, Saudi Arabia, Dubai, England, and more. I have always wished that as a family we could go on an oversees trip to see how the other half of the world lives, but if that's not fiscally feasible, then God sure found a creative way to bring the world to us!

In the words of one of our recent stranger-turned-friends:

"Not only did we sing, but we also danced and had big laughs with a big family in a big, big world. We are all here as internationals, and the world is getting smaller. The world got smaller in our hands in this wonderful house tonight."

Sometimes we think that we want to be with people just like us, but I would rather have a quilt on my bed then a solid colored blanket any day. The tapestry of life that God designed in the human heart fascinates me to no end. Behind every patch on the quilt, every new face, is a breath-taking story. God fearfully and wonderfully made each one of us.

"We want to raise our children so that they can take a sense of pleasure in both their own heritage and the diversity of others."

~ Mr. Rogers

If it's good enough for Mr. Rogers, it's good enough for me. By the way, with 35 people, we did cook two turkeys!

How can you take the initiative to be more outgoing in your workplace? School? Home? Place of worship? Neighborhood? City? World?

STA5GE

Continuation

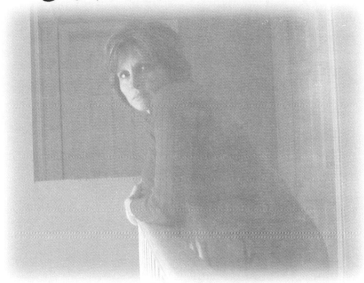

"Don't let it faze you.
Stick with what you learned and believed."

(The Message)

Too Early to Quit

"You have to forget your last marathon before you try another. Your mind can't know what's coming."
~ Frank Shorter

Have you ever run a marathon before? Continuation in the journey is so difficult and critical. If you don't continue for the duration of the 26.2 miles, then you won't reach your finish line.

Thus far, I have run 11 marathons total with the Detroit Free Press/Flagstar Marathon, the Dallas White Rock Marathon, and the Martian Marathon. Detroit and Dallas were obviously both city marathons, with music and spectators to cheer on the runners. The Martian Marathon was the total opposite. The Martian course was along Hines Drive – a long, peaceful, tree-lined road with minimal streetlights and little traffic. An occasional park can be seen, but it's relatively stimulus-free and runner friendly.

While the Martian Marathon is one I'd highly recommend, the course was mentally tough for me. Within the first two miles, my mind was completely shocked by the tranquil setting with its natural beauty. I had been so used to the festivities and music in the city marathons, but there were no bands playing along Hines Drive. Few high-fives greeted me along the way, and certainly no one was holding up any signs for me. "How could I continue like this?" I questioned.

"It's always too early to quit."
~ Vincent Peale

When was the last time you found yourself "stuck" in a situation? That's just how I felt at mile two. (If you do the math that means I had 24.2 demanding miles to go. Yikes!) My self-talk went like this, "Lisa, what have you gotten yourself in to? Do you realize that all of these trees look the same? (Perhaps I should have imagined them as people cheering me on!) Green may be your favorite color, but this is green overload. Green, green, and more green. Can you really stand looking at 26.2 miles worth of trees? HOW are you going to make this with little outside support (also known as distractions)?"

"Running is a big question mark that's there each and every day. It asks you, 'Are you going to be a wimp or are you going to be strong today?'"
~ Peter Maher, Irish-Canadian Olympian
and Sub-2:12 marathoner

Around mile five (which felt like mile 15), a jolly fellow ran along side me. Long distance runners are a rare breed unto themselves, so I didn't think too much about his comments, until he told me with all sincerity that he was going to actually win this race. "Oh, really?" I asked, quickly reasoning that if this guy is running with me, he is definitely not going to be winning any races! Then I thought, *Oh, Lord. Am I going to be stuck running next to this guy the whole way?* Between looking at the sea of trees and listening to my gabby, over-confident companion, I really believed I might have a mental breakdown. For the first time in a long time, I wondered how I was going to continue. Can you relate?

"What matters is not necessarily the size of the dog in the fight – it's the size of the fight in the dog."
~ Dwight D. Eisenhower

Fortunately, at mile seven I tactfully pulled away from my jovial friend. Next came Craig, a 50-year-old ultra marathoner who had run one marathon in every state. That's 50 marathons! I figured that the likelihood of Craig maintaining our pace and actually finishing was quite high, so I stayed close to him like a bee docs to honey. While conversing and running we tried to solve the world's problems, and the miles just seemed to fly by.

Something else stood out to me when I ran with Craig. What seemed like happenstance turned out to be a fascinating exchange. I found out that he was a card-carrying atheist. Craig did most of the talking while we ran. I chose to do most of the listening. He wasn't use to a Christian who would listen more than she talked! I think he appreciated this. At the end of this Martian Marathon we gave each other a warm, sweaty, and genuine hug. "Who said Christians and atheists can't be friends?" I asked. To my sheer delight, our friendship continued. The following summer Craig and his lovely wife, Connie, entertained all of the Harpers at their gorgeous, lakefront home in Minnesota. We tubed on their lake to our hearts' content. What a blast! I must say that Craig and Connie rank as some of the finest hosts we've ever met. It's amazing where the marathon of life takes us, isn't it?

What a difference a friend can make – even new friends! Which friends in your life have come along side that help you continue? Today, who can you help to continue in their race of life?

Life is a Highway

"The ant is knowing and wise,
but he doesn't know enough to take a vacation."
~ Clarence Day

What in the world do vacations have to do with continuation? Isn't a vacation a respite, a type of halting from the mundane? Exactly. Taking vacations will help us continue in this marathon called life. If we don't put forth the effort and planning, a lack of vacations can be a recipe for burn out. Burn out can cause bail out, and God may not want us to bail out just yet! By taking even the simplest of vacations, we can regain our strength and stamina.

What were some of your favorite childhood vacations? For the Fourth of July, I frequently enjoyed driving with my parents to Bessemer in the Upper Peninsula of Michigan. I'll also never forget the 24-hour trek from Michigan to Florida with my mother and brother Jeff.

When our Harper children were younger, we visited a quaint cottage on a quiet lake in Pullman, Michigan. The lake was shallow for the children, and the fishing was easy for the novice. We had loads of fun when we got there, but getting there was a whole other story.

"A vacation frequently means that the family goes
away for a rest, accompanied by a mother
who sees that the others get it."
~ Marcelene Cox

All of the packing, the diapers (when the kids were younger), the food, the towels, the sunscreen, the shoes (hopefully in pairs), the right clothes for every person, trip paraphernalia, and of course, the dog. It's no wonder we needed a full-sized van!

"Those that say you can't take it with you
never saw a car packed for a vacation trip."
~ Anonymous

Sometimes I have wondered if it's truly worth it to break from the routine. Is that really a vacation? It may not be the same as going on a romantic cruise with my Sweety, but the answer is still yes.

"Vacation is what you take when you can't take
what you've been taking any longer."
~ Adeline Ainsworth

Our family road trips have taken us thousands of highway miles. We have driven from Detroit to Halifax, St. Louis, Nashville, Washington D.C., Boston, Little Rock, Tulsa, Chicago, Minneapolis, the Apostle Islands of Lake Superior, and even the Smokey Mountains. Twice we attempted to drive somewhere warm during the winter, only to be forced to wear our parkas while strolling along the Gulf Coast beach in Florida and the Atlantic Ocean beach of North Carolina. Who wants to drive over one thousand miles to wear a parka when I can just step out my front door in Michigan and wear one? Not me, but all of those trips were so worth it.

My favorite place to vacation is the shores of Lake Michigan along the Sleeping Bear Dunes. I love the water and beach. I love to feel the fine sand between my toes and the rumbling rocks under my soles. I love surfing the waves and soaking in the sunsets. I love running along the barrier-free beach for miles, with no agenda chasing after me.

Our family vacations pay huge dividends in the long run (no pun intended)! Our daily schedules are altered. We wake up randomly. We eat unique foods and see new places. We even play "Apples to Apples" more than normal and eat twice as many freshly-baked, chocolate chip cookies as should be legal. In addition, many of those vacations are cell phone-TV-and computer-free. What? No checking emails for a week? That's right. My emails don't own me. I own my emails.

All good things must come to an end, including vacations. But somehow, magically, at the end of my favorite vacations I have a new-found energy to face a new tomorrow. When was the last time you took a vacation you enjoyed? What can you do to make it happen again?

Happy Birthday to You

"Middle age is when you choose your cereal
for the fiber, not the toy."
~ Unknown

Do you remember your favorite cereal as a child? Mine was Cocoa Puffs (with a striped yo-yo inside). On one special occasion, my Uncle Tim took my brother Jeff and me to Rush Lake in Atlanta, Michigan, for some one-on-one time. Uncle Tim was like the perfect uncle who would engage us in camping, canoeing and even concerts. As only a cool uncle would do, he let us eat Cocoa Puffs for breakfast, lunch and dinner for two days in a row! Who wouldn't want an uncle like that?

In addition to sugarcoated cereals with tempting toys inside, children are known to love birthdays. Each birthday marks another year of life, and that truly calls for celebration. In the case of the Harpers, that means a mammoth birthday cake loaded with layers of Oreo cookie crust, ice cream, chocolate sauce, and whip cream. Delicious!

For most adults, however, there comes a point in our lives when we lose the excitement about continuous birthdays. How do *you* feel when your birthday rolls around?

"It's so sad to grow old alone.
My wife hasn't had a birthday in four years.
She was born in the year of our Lord-only-knows."
~ Anonymous

Why is it that when we are young we want to grow up, and when we are old we want to go back?

Even the wisest philosophers, scholars, and scientists can't hold back time, and why should they? I'm a firm believer that each day is a gift from God, and age is, in some respects, a matter of the mind. If we continue to move our bodies to the extent that we are personally able, we *can* slow down the aging process!

I have never witnessed an adult age as gracefully as my timeless gymnastics coach, Frances Borgo. Frances looked the same to me for about 30 years. She could do a commercial for Noxema with ease. I used to think, *What is it with Frances? She is amazing!* It was no secret to the thousands of students that had Frances as a teacher (during her seven decades of teaching) what kept Frances young for life: She exercised daily; Frances swam, danced, walked, stretched, ate well, laughed, smiled, prayed, and kept a positive attitude. Sure, she must have had challenging days, but she never wore her problems on her sleeve. When I grow up, I want to be just like Frances!

"In the end, it's not the years in your life that count,
but the life in your years."
~ Abraham Lincoln

I know that I'm getting older when I forget how old I am! Has that ever happened to you? I also have "senior moments," and I'm not even a senior yet. Now that's frightening. Yet, who says we have to fear growing old or even lie about it? There's no reason to be embarrassed. Embrace the age that you are. You can't turn back the clock, but you sure can slow it down. It's never too late to replace unhealthy habits with better ones. As for me, don't ever tell me that you can't teach this old dog a few new tricks.

Cocoa Puffs won't stop the aging of our bodies (or the continuation of birthdays), but a few other factors might. What steps can you take today to remain (or become) young in body, mind, and spirit? You really can do it. Happy Birthday to YOU!

"The older the fiddler, the sweeter the tune."
~ Pope Paul VI

Land Ho

"You've got to get up every morning with determination if you are going to go to bed every night with satisfaction."

~ George Lorimer

*H*ave you ever started something that you didn't finish? Perhaps it was a house project half done, a room half painted, a book half read, a business goal left hanging, a scarf half knit, a lawn half mowed, an office half organized, or even a bed half made!

To initiate any activity requires effort. To continue through the process until it is completed requires tremendous resolve. History proves this well:

Bury a person in the snows of Valley Forge, and you have a George Washington. Raise him in abject poverty, and you have an Abraham Lincoln. Strike him down with infantile paralysis, and he becomes a Franklin D. Roosevelt. Burn him so severely that the doctors say he will never walk again, and you have Glenn Cunningham, who set the world's one-mile record in 1934...Call him a slow learner and retarded...writing him off as uneducable, and you have an Albert Einstein.

~ John Maxwell

Another historical hero is Christopher Columbus. Can you imagine what would have happened if Columbus had not continued his renowned, risky voyage across the Atlantic in 1492? The journey was fierce on numerous fronts, and Columbus was given ample reasons to quit. After a few weeks of sailing westward, Columbus writes in his log of an anxious crew full of impatience and fear. They had witnessed a falling meteorite and tall weeds that seemed to almost swallow them alive. Moreover, seeing their north compass move nearly put them over the edge – literally! Those poor sailors begged Columbus to return to Spain before their food ran out, or a mysterious sea creature would eat them. They feared they would sail off the edge of their world and fall into the Sea of Darkness.

When was the last time you felt like you were approaching a Sea of Darkness? It may not be easy, but let's take a lesson from Columbus and continue to courageously sail on.

> *"I am . . . confident that if I lose command,*
> *the fleet will never reach the Indies*
> *and will probably never get back to Spain.*
> *With God's help I shall persevere."*
> ~ Christopher Columbus

Knowing full well of the plans of mutiny and sabotage, Columbus wrote in two sets of logs. One log was kept private, showing the true distance that they had sailed from shore. The second log was made public in the hopes of calming the sailors. This log under-reported the true distance traveled. In this way, Columbus reasoned that the crew would feel more secure being closer to home. In spite of their plethora of struggles, he ended each day by recording this in his log:

"Today we sailed westward."
~ Christopher Columbus

By December 10 of 1492, Columbus promised his crews of the Nina, Pinta, and Santa Maria that if they did not see land in two days, then they would return home. Much to everyone's peace of mind, they saw land the next day. If it had not been for the faith, determination, and perseverance of Columbus the admiral, we might not have America as we know it today. Thankfully, Columbus and his sailors finished what they started.

What have you put off finishing? Have you listened to discouraging voices for too long? Today is your day to take that goal off the shelf and continue where you left off. Fix your eyes on the prize at the finish line. Picture yourself continuing strong to the end. Go ahead. Finish that book. Paint that room. Write that business plan. Both you and God will know that you *did* accomplish something worthwhile. Find your true north in life, and sail on. Your "land ho" may be just around the corner.

"A ship in harbor is safe –
but that is not what ships are for."
~ John A. Shedd

Which Butter is Better?

*C*an you read this tongue-twisting rhyme out loud? Try to say it continuously from beginning to end!

Betty Botter

Betty Botter bought some butter,
But, she said, the butter's bitter.
If I put it in my batter,
It will make my batter bitter.
But a bit of better butter
Is sure to make my batter better.
So she bought a bit of butter
Better than her bitter butter
And she put it in her batter
And the batter was not bitter
So 'twas better Betty Botter
Bought a bit of better butter.

That's quite a collection of words. Looking at the simple meaning of the message, you'll see that Betty bought some bitter butter, which did not work out so great. So she bought some better butter, which seemed to do the trick. Here's a question for you: Who do you think taught her how to buy the better butter? I venture to guess that it was probably her parents!

Being a parent who educates is one of the most humbling roles in the world. As parents, we are responsible for the physical, social, emotional, spiritual, and intellectual well being of our children. No pressure, right? Wrong! There is a ton of pressure, but with God's help, we can do it.

"Children are not casual guests in our home. They have been loaned to us temporarily for the purpose of loving them and instilling a foundation of values on which their future lives will be built."
~ Dr. James Dobson

In terms of our children's educational needs, Scott and I believe that the oversight is still our obligation, no matter where they go to school. Teaching our children is a continual, life-long process. As parents, we are instructing all the time, whether we realize it or not. Now isn't *that* a scary thought?

Fortunately, education is one of my passions, having majored in elementary education in college. By the time our oldest daughter Autumn was born, I had already finished a master's degree in reading from Eastern Michigan University. During a five-year period of time, I enjoyed tutoring more than 40 students in our home. Our children grew up surrounded by the joy of learning (most of the time!), so it's no surprise that at the age of two, Autumn asked, "Mommy, will you tutor me?"

"Well, of course!" I responded. So this school teacher became a private tutor who became a home-school teacher. What a great fit! I poured my heart and soul into Autumn, Jonathan, Victoria, and Jasmine while they were at home. Attending RECESS, an outstanding homeschool co-op in the Detroit area, exposed each of them to wonderful teachers, curriculum, activities, and values-centered families. My kids thrived on the creativity of it all!

*"People rarely succeed unless they have fun
in what they are doing."*
~ Dale Carnegie

Throughout the years, the methods of education have continually changed for the Harpers. We've done it all - home school, Christian school, and public school. At times I had an internal agenda, but I quickly realized that I needed to treat each of my children as unique individuals and seek God's will for every one of them every year.

Did you know that God's plan is always best, and it often requires us to adapt our pre-conceived wishes to His better ways? Through our family's educational changes, I have learned to trust God more.

What's the best way for you to teach your children to buy the best butter? Ask God to show you, and continue full steam ahead!

"Point your kids in the right direction.
When they are old they won't be lost."
~ Proverbs 22:6 (The Message)

STAGE 6

Obstruction

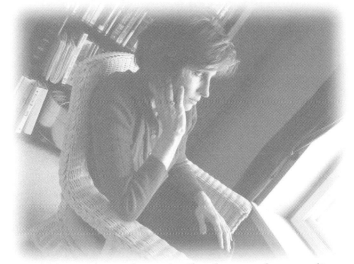

"Why are you down in the dumps, dear soul?
Why are you crying the blues?
Fix my eyes on God—
soon I'll be praising again.
He puts a smile on my face.
He's my God."

(The Message)

Scaling the Wall

"Never again," I declared to the world after running a 3:09 marathon at the 1985 Detroit Free Press/Flagstar Marathon. "I will never again run another 26.2 miles." For some reason, I was convinced that in order for me to run another one, I would need to do it even faster!

"Never let the fear of striking out get in your way."
~ George Herman "Babe" Ruth

How could I run any faster? I wondered. I knew the cross-training regimen I underwent to run that fast: running 60-70 miles per week, swimming a mile three times a week, plus occasional gymnastics. With such a variety of physical fitness activities, I flourished. During college, working out twice a day was so much fun for me. For some people, this would be torture!

*"Exercise is a dirty word. Every time I hear it,
I wash my mouth out with chocolate."*
~ Charles Shulz

For 17 years (and through the changes that came from being a wife, gymnastics coach, tutor, teacher, pastor's wife, and mother who had been pregnant nine times) I put my "marathoner hat" on the shelf. "Nope. It's not in the cards for me," I accepted. Yet, after our youngest was born, I took full advantage of no more pregnancies (translation: no more rubber band mama)! I began to run two to three miles, a few times a week. Even though I felt like I was starting from scratch, I craved getting into the running again.

"There is no such thing as a long piece of work, except one that you dare not start."
~ Charles Baudelaire

Gone was the faulty assumption that in order for me to run another marathon, I must break my PR (personal record.) I was just having the time of my life lacing up my shoes again and feeling the breeze blow through my hair! Gradually, I increased my running to four to five miles at a crack, four to five times a week.

Extra! Extra! Read all about it! It was a Monday in October of 2002 when I read this full page spread in the Detroit Free Press Newspaper: *"Run! Run! Run!"* Instantly, those words cried out to me; I had a newfound desire to run a full marathon (26.2 miles) once more. However, there was just one major obstruction: the marathon was six days away!

While I would not recommend this to anyone, I actually ran the Detroit marathon six days later. I had done zero…nada…zilch…no long training runs in 17 years. When I told Scott of my wild idea on that Monday, he could have responded, "No way, Lisa! You are out of your mind." But instead he lovingly exhorted me: "Lisa, if it would be fun for you, then you should do it. But if you need to walk or stop, that's okay." Gratefully, my courageous husband allowed me to pursue this short-sighted, huge-hearted goal. How breath-taking (in more ways than one!)

> *"Keep away from people who try to belittle*
> *your ambitions. Small people always do that,*
> *but the really great make you feel that*
> *you, too, can become great."*
> ~ Mark Twain

During that marathon I actually ran to mile 22 without walking! Then I "hit the wall," thereby walking and jogging the rest of the way. That was fine with me. I knew my kamikaze marathon was a crazy attempt. But I did it with a smile!

What obstructions hinder you from running your race of life? Do you have a "crazy" goal you've been putting off because you lack the encouragement? Not every wall is a permanent barrier. Some walls are meant to climb over – and conquer!

> *"With my God I can scale a wall!"*
> ~ II Samuel 22:30 (The Message)

The Miracle of Life

"Raising children is like making biscuits:
it is as easy to raise a big batch as one,
while you have your hands in the dough."
~ E.W. Howe

What one word would people use to describe you? For me, it might be "Italian" because of my deep affection for children. I always desired a large family to recreate the best-friend scenario that exists between my older siblings and me. Can you picture your fondest childhood memories?

I remember when my sister Julie put my sleepy body into a bed with dirty, chop suey pans. She wanted to see my twinkle toes mix with the rice and vegetables. Or the times when teenage Tom would yell and beat his chest like Tarzan, jumping from balconies in our Sherwood Forest neighborhood. Or when Mark, the budding artist, drew all over my face (with black, permanent marker) while I was sleeping. Or the time when Jeff fed me raw, soggy French toast, claiming that it was really cooked!

"Having children is like having a bowling alley
installed in your brain."
~ Alan Bleasdale

111

Together we laughed. Together we cried. I often thought that the best gift that my parents gave me was my siblings. After Scott and I were married in 1986, I wanted to provide that same joy for my offspring.

Little did I expect that I would have numerous fertility issues. Before our oldest daughter, Autumn, was born, I had three miscarriages. The first time I was in shock. The second time I was angry. By the third time, I was just plain sad.

Have you ever wanted something so badly, you would do whatever it took to get it? The miscarriages were a huge obstruction to our desire for a large family, and there was nothing I could do about it. I even stopped running and was cautious to do everything right. Nothing seemed to help, or so I thought.

Just when I almost gave up, God gave us three wonderful children in four years: Autumn, Jonathan, and Victoria. During Victoria's birthing process, the umbilical cord was wrapped around her neck. Prayers went up quickly. God answered those prayers in such a mighty way that the nurse told the doctor of a supernatural intervention that occurred in the delivery room. Victoria was born victorious! When it rains, it pours. Our quiver felt almost full.

"Making the decision to have a child is momentous.
It is to decide forever to have your heart
go walking around outside your body."
~ Elizabeth Stone

While I was exceedingly grateful for the children we had, I believed that God created another one to complete our family. But next, I had two more miscarriages. By the fifth miscarriage, my heart was forlorn. I felt like I was on the operating table for open-heart surgery, and no one was sewing me up! For pregnancy number nine, I petitioned God to either take the conviction away or make it happen. (Did you know that even optimistic people like me still suffer?) In my mind, whatever the outcome, that was going to be my last pregnancy.

Before you were conceived I wanted you.
Before you were born I loved you.
Before you were here an hour I would die for you.
This is the miracle of life.
~ Maureen Hawkins

God is never late and never early – He's always on time. When our Jasmine Rose was born, I declared with a smile and a sigh of relief, "It is finished!" Our Harper family had the exclamation point at the end of our sentence. God was and is faithful!

Don't let your obstructions have the final say. You and I can get bitter (like that bitter butter a few stories ago) or we can say, "I don't understand it all, but I will trust you, Lord." When you are at the end of your rope, where do you turn?

"What we do with what we don't understand
is just as important as what we do
with what we do understand."
~ Bill Johnson

Blue Days and Blue Skies

Blue days, all of them gone.
Nothin' but blue skies from now on.
Blue skies smilin' at me.
Nothin' but blue skies do I see.
~ Bing Crosby

*W*ho doesn't want blue skies instead of blue days? In the hit 1950s' musical classic, *White Christmas*, Bing Crosby led a star-studded cast, including Rosemary Clooney, Danny Kaye and Vera Ellen, in one of the most beloved Christmas movies of all time. The four of them finished the movie by putting on a surprise show for a needy, retired army general at his desolate lodge. At the end, the softhearted general was blessed to have his former troops show up (in old uniforms a little too tight for their tummies) for the music and dancing gig. To top it off, their Vermont setting was finally graced with a timely snowfall on that Christmas Eve – making it the White Christmas they had all been dreaming of.

Have all of your Christmases been white? I'm not just talking "snowy." I'm talking happy. I wish that I could say that all of our Harper Christmases were figuratively white (with blue skies to match), but one Christmas time definitely wasn't.

What comes to your mind when you think of Christmas? When I think of Christmas time, I think of floods of festive presents, shimmering lights, colorful cards, and Christmas carols. I look forward to Grandma Kathy's cookies, Grandpa Nutt's chili, Grandpa Rick's coffee, Grandma Glory's French toast sticks, and Grandmother Anne Harper's Christmas Eve dinners. What I don't expect is a flood of water in our basement on the Sunday morning before Christmas! What a depressing and untimely obstruction!

Sunday mornings for a pastor's family are chalked full of multi-tasking opportunities. On this particular Sunday morning, adorned in my festive Christmas dress and nylons, I walked into our basement office to print out a Christmas flyer. Splish, splash, my feet were suddenly taking a bath.

*"Only a fool tests the depth of the water
with both feet."*
~ African proverb

Unfortunately, we had experienced two basement floods before, so I knew what the culprit was: the sump pump. My stocking feet were soaked, and the freshly flowing water was seeping into my long-hemmed Christmas dress. Pencils and pictures were floating everywhere. With a gasp I almost collapsed and cried, but it was a busy Sunday morning; I didn't have time to feel sorry for myself. (That came later!) My husband had already been at First Assembly for hours, and I was home alone with the four children.

"We cannot continue to lurch from one disaster to another. There are people who have been hit with severe flooding three times in the last five years."
~ Robert Brady

I quickly awakened all four children and pulled them into the hallway. We had this heavy heart-to-heart conversation:

"You guys… the basement flooded again," I told them.

"What? It flooded *again*?" they asked, with jaw-dropping disbelief.

"Yes," I calmly replied. "Autumn, I know you just got your license, but you need to be the mom right now and drive our van to church. Please play the piano in my place. Jonathan, you still play drums. Victoria and Jasmine, please help with children's church. I'll stay here and work on this."

Then we said a prayer together. I wanted to model to our kids what they can do in the future when they face obstacles: turn to God for help. At that moment, we purposefully made Him our "center." He helped us regroup in the weeks ahead, and the six of us even painted portions of the basement…together!

What do you do when tragedy hits your family? Do you rely upon yourself or rely upon God? Sooner or later, with God as your center, your blue days will turn into blue skies!

How's Your CORE Strength?

*"Count the garden by the flowers,
never by the leaves that fall. Count your life
with smiles and not the tears that roll."*
~ Anonymous

Do you look at your life like a glass that's half empty or half full? Are you counting your flowers or the leaves that fall? John Maxwell says, "Your attitude determines your altitude." I couldn't agree more. It's not uncommon for people to use the hardships in their lives as excuses for their current conditions. While I am sure there is truly some cause and effect, I also realize that we all make choices in life, too. It's easier for us to blame others than to take appropriate responsibility ourselves.

Have you ever played the blame game? I have. As a runner, I blamed the heat and humidity for a poor 10K performance at the Oak Apple Run, when in reality I just wasn't in very good shape. We blame the dog for "chewing our homework," when in reality, we just didn't finish it. Sometimes in this competitive race of life, soccer parents blame the coaches when perhaps their child wasn't as prepared for the game as he or she should have been. We even blame the weatherman for the weather.

119

For Scott and me, we could easily look at our childhood years through the lenses of shame and blame. Between the two of us, there were five divorces among our parents. During the 1960s, it was rare in our educational and social circles to be raised by a single parent like we were. Primarily his dad, Mark Harper, raised Scott and his three older brothers (Clark, Mark, and Fred). In comparison, primarily my mother, Donna Cummings, raised the five of us (Tom, Mark, Julie, Jeff, and yours truly). When I was five years old, I remember my parents calling all of the children into the living room. My mother and father were wonderful people, yet they told us that they were getting a divorce. I didn't know what that was, but I just knew that it was really bad. I started crying.

"Those who sow with tears
will reap with songs of joy."
~ Psalm 126:5 (NIV)

Unlike most divorced families, however, Scott and I both stayed in close contact with our other loving, biological parent. By a miracle of God, all of our current biological parents and their mates (on both sides) get along very well. We even have periodic holidays together. Can you picture this? Grandpa Rick Donovan strums his guitar while bellowing John Denver songs. Grandmother Anne Harper strokes the piano keys with the likes of Mozart and Chopin. (Not at the exact same time as Grandpa Rick, but yes, in the same evening!)

While our upbringings weren't exactly like *Leave It to Beaver*, Scott and I have always experienced significant parental support on all fronts. For example, when I was a teenager I was in my first car accident on 8 Mile Road in Detroit. Unfortunately, I was not driving a clunker of a car. I was driving my father's new Honda Accord. (How many of you parents would allow your teenager to drive your new car around town, within days of the purchase? That shows you the trust factor of my openhanded, level-headed father, Tom Nutt.) When the accident happened, I cried huge tears and just felt terrible. My father could have really gotten upset with me, particularly since he was supposed to drive his new car to Chicago the next day!

Instead, my father sat next to me, took my hand, and encouraged me with these words: "Lisa, the car is just a thing. You are more important than the car. Now don't you worry. We can get the car fixed. I'm just glad that you weren't hurt."

His response was so comforting and therapeutic. I was also quite impressed that this successful businessman was willing to be seen in public driving west for over three hundred miles, in a mangled auto with a disfigured front end.

Thankfully, most of my childhood memories are fond ones. Nevertheless, all of these divorces in our families had the potential to be monumental obstructions. Once Scott and I got married, who were we supposed to look to as a strong Christian model for marriage and family? It certainly wouldn't be Hollywood. We could have used the divorces as an excuse to be stuck in our ways and not strive to thrive in our marriage, but we didn't.

"Depression loses its power
when fresh vision pierces the darkness."
~ Peter Sinclair

"The buck stops here!" we declared. Enough already – no more divorces! We can't control what's been done in the past, but we can control our own marital destiny. "Let's have a faith-vision for *our* marriage and make it the best it can be…but how?"

Practically speaking, Dr. Dobson (Focus on the Family) recommends CORE, an acrostic highlighting a terrific four-step intimacy process for making marriages strong: Commitment, Openness, Repentance, and Empathy.

Today can be a fresh start for your family. When was the last time you dated your mate? What improvements can be made to strengthen the CORE of your marriage? Your whole family is worth this investment – and generations to come will thank you for it!

Music Therapy

*P*icture the most fearful experience of your life. Was it riding on the world's tallest and fastest roller coaster, Top Thrill Dragster, at Cedar Point? What about giving a persuasive speech or starting a new job? Fear can also be described with the acrostic False Evidence Appearing Real.

When was a fear real to you, but it wasn't really true? A few years back I experienced unwarranted fear that gave me deep empathy for those who suffer with mental illness. I had a serious hamstring injury and was instructed by a sports medicine specialist to get a MRI (Magnetic Resonance Imaging) test. "No problem," I reasoned. "I'll just lay there while they can take a few painless pictures."

My MRI took place at a high-caliber university in Michigan. I was actually looking forward to the "laying down" part, because I thought it would be a wonderful opportunity for Hurricane Lisa to slow down a bit. So, I lay on the slightly concave table, with a dandy beeper in hand. "If you want to stop this 45-minute process, or you need to come out for any reason," directed the technician, "just press this button."

Sure thing, but why would I need this button if I'm just resting on the table? In addition, why would I want to stop the process? It's completely pain free. We need these results for physical therapy. After all, I did want to run another marathon soon.

"Now I lay me down to sleep.
I pray the Lord my soul to keep.
If I die before I wake,
I pray the Lord my soul to take."
~ 18th Century Children's Prayer

"Crank. Crank." All of a sudden, the firm, slender bed I was "resting" on became like a tray. I was sliding right into the oven of fear, feet first! It wasn't so bad when my eyes still saw daylight, but when my whole body squished into that tube, I thought I was going to have a nervous breakdown! I felt claustrophobic. The tray moved in further with a series of jerks. Remember, I was supposed to lie completely still so that the technicians could get the most accurate pictures. *We wouldn't want to have to do this whole thing over again now, would we?*

"Beep. Beep." My nimble fingers pressed on that alarm button quicker than a cat can catch a mouse, and the ladies pulled the tray out of the oven. My heart was racing much faster than it ever does in a marathon. With determination I sat up and told those lovely ladies a thing or two: "Oh, no. I'm not going back in there. I know that you need these test results, but I'm telling you right now that you are going to have to KNOCK...ME...OUT!"

"There are very few monsters
who warrant the fear we have of them."
~ Andre Gide

The nurses proceeded to tell me how they had nice medicine that would calm me down and help me slide back into the forbidden chambers. "No way!" I insisted. "I am a very smart person, and mind altering drugs aren't going to do it for me!" At that defining moment, I became a high maintenance patient. (In hindsight, if I could have brought Grandpa Rick's guitar music into the chamber, that might have helped! He has a way of lifting almost anyone's heavy heart.)

Thanks be to God, a few weeks later, I had an "open-aired" MRI. Listening to faith-filled Psalms* with peaceful piano music in the background (also known as music therapy) helped me overcome the phobia. God's Word was the *only means* of bringing comfort to my soul.

How do you handle fear? Have you read a Psalm* or two lately? It's better than milk and does a body good!

* Book of the Bible, found in the Old Testament

STAGE 7

Anticipation

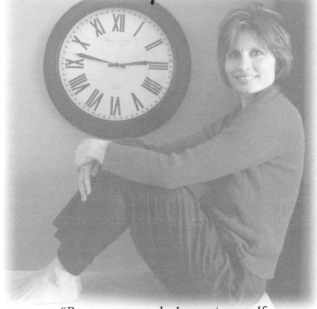

"By no means do I count myself
an expert in all of this,
but I've got my eye on the goal,
where God is beckoning us onward…
I'm off and running, and I'm not turning back."

(The Message)

See the End from the Beginning

"If you set a goal for yourself and are able to achieve it, you have won your race. Your goal can be to come in first, to improve your performance, or just to finish the race – it's up to you."

~ Dave Scott

*O*ut of all the aspects of a marathon, I anticipate the start and the finish the most. The night before a marathon I can hardly sleep. While resting on my pillow, I picture the entire marathon route in my head and visualize myself finishing strong. I anticipate it. I even salivate over it! My goal is to finish the marathon *running*, and to run the whole way without stopping once. (It's just a practice I have while running my marathons.)

"Even if you are on the right track,
you'll get run over if you just sit there."
~ Will Rogers

What is it like to be at the starting line of a marathon? It is electrifying! My adrenaline is pumping and my heart is thumping. I love to hear the music fill the air. People cheer and wave to runners as if we are movie stars. Where else in life do so many strangers cheer each other on?

At some point along the route, I mentally wish that I could merely skip the remaining miles and magically arrive at the finish. Isn't it that way in life? When have you longed to gracefully exit out of a circumstance and immediately find yourself in a better one?

"Winning isn't always finishing first.
Sometimes winning is just finishing."
~ Manuel Diotte

There are always humorous marathon moments that get my mind off of the pain. I see runners dressed up as flags, presidents, sports stars, and more. I meet funny dudes, sassy divas, super heroes, and even outer-space aliens. They talk about topics like the weather, football, jobs, family, vacations, running routes, and even food!

"My therapist told me the way to achieve
true inner peace is to finish what I start.
So far today, I have finished two bags of M&Ms
and a chocolate cake. I feel better already."
~ Dave Barry

Do you know what I anticipate the very most about my marathons with Marathon Mission? I can hardly wait to cross the finish line; I check on the status of our team. Who made it, and who's still "on the track?" When any Marathon Mission team member is still pounding the pavement, I truly wish that I could go back on the course and run along side them to help them finish. In fact, if it wasn't against the rules, I would do just that!

A few years ago at the Seattle Special Olympics, nine contestants, all physically or mentally disabled, assembled at the starting line for the 100-yard dash. At the gun they all started out, not exactly in a dash, but with the relish to run the race to the finish and win. All, that is, except one boy who stumbled on the asphalt, tumbled over a couple of times, and began to cry. The other eight heard the boy cry. They slowed down and paused. Then they all turned around and went back. Every one of them. One girl with Down's syndrome bent down and kissed him and said, "This will make it better." Then all nine linked arms and walked together to the finish line. Everyone in the stadium stood, and the cheering went on for 10 minutes.

~ Anonymous

When have you demonstrated endurance? What has helped you cross your finish line? How can you help others do the same?

Standing for the Chorus

"Life is one grand, sweet song…so start the music."
~ Ronald Reagan

*M*usic is a powerful motivator – a "Big Mo." Which tunes propel you or soothe your soul? When I need to clean, I turn on, *Celebrate Good Times.* To lift a heavy heart, I listen to, *Healer.* The Charlie Brown theme song makes me smile. Moreover, when our family needs a "pick-me-up," we bellow, *The Sun Will Come Out…Tomorrow* from Annie.

"Some people come into our lives, leave footprints on our hearts, and we are never the same."
~ Franz Schubert

Was there someone significant in your life who imparted music (or another gift) into you? My musical roots can be traced back to a tremendous piano teacher in her 80s, Mary Klein. In her hey day, she played 40-page songs for the Detroit Symphony Orchestra…by memory. I was her very last pupil. Mrs. Klein *anticipated* that something good was going to come of her efforts. Consequently, she would freely and passionately give me 90-minute lessons of intense classical training.

"Too many people die
with their music still inside them."
~ Oscar Wilde

Other musicians who refused to die "with their music still inside them" were my grandmother Evelyn and great aunts Gertie, Bea, and Betty Vaillancourt. They sang and danced in Vaudeville in the 1920s and 1930s. Known for their humorous ways, natural talent, and tight harmonies, they passed on the traditions to my melodious mother, Donna. She would sing to soothe and entertain all of us with lyrics like, "Shoe fly pie, and apple pandowdy – You never get enough of that wonderful stuff!" How true! I wish I could live in the harmonies of life 24/7. Don't you?

Has someone ever sung or played an instrument for you? How did that make you feel? There is no piece of music that moves me more than Handel's *Messiah*.

Such public inspiration for the *Messiah* began centuries ago. George Frederick Handel first performed his *Messiah* in 1742 in Dublin, Ireland. In fact, Handel was inspired to compose oratorios like this one because many citizens of the day could not read or afford a Bible. Thus, Handel put powerful, compelling Scriptures about Christ to music so those listeners would learn the hope of God's Word. How Handel was able to sketch and score the entire *Messiah*, full of drama and pathos, in three weeks is truly beyond comprehension.

*"Whether I was in my body or out of my body
as I wrote it I know not. God knows."*
~ George Handel

Have you had the pleasure of witnessing Handel's *Messiah* performed live? If so, I'm certain that the audience stood for the highly anticipated "Hallelujah Chorus." Why the standing? History tells us that King George II of England was so inspired when hearing the chorus that he stood. When the king stood, the audience also rose. That tradition still remains.

My favorite part is the crescendo: "And He shall reign forever and ever. King of Kings and Lord of Lords. Halle-lu-jah!" Part of me cries out, "Just take me to heaven right now! This must be what it's like!"

*"The aim and final end of all music should be
none other than the glory of God and the
refreshment of the soul."*
~ Johan Sebastian Bach

Today, what melody is playing on the strings of your heart? When you were born, God stood up to cheer the lifesong of *you*. He's still standing for you today, with unceasing anticipation…cheering you on in your race of life. What's your greatest expectation? The sun *will* come out tomorrow. With God, the best is yet to come!

Lost and Found

*"After the tone, leave your name, number, and tell
where you left the money. I'll get back to you as
soon as it's safe for you to come out of hiding."*
~ Anonymous

*W*hen was the last time you played hide and seek?
When our children were younger, they loved to
play hide and seek with each other. They'd hide in
cramped nooks and crannies - under beds and inside
cupboards. (We could have done without the "hiding
in the drier" bit.) Once, we noticed something hilarious: All of them were hiding, and no one was seeking!

*"The spring has sprung, the grass is rizz.
I wonder where them birdies is?"*
~ Winnie the Pooh

Even as adults, we play hide and seek all of the time. Is
it just me, or as we age and as we seek, do we forget
where we put items of value?

*"I have the answer in my head.
I just haven't found it yet."*
~ Anonymous

Personally, I have a difficult time remembering the passwords, logins, and user ID's for important computer Web sites. How frustrating! Okay, for those of you who are logical, I understand the realities of identity theft and the importance of Internet security, but how is the average person like me supposed to remember which "codes" I need for what – particularly if the secret codes are case sensitive? The codes become so secretive that I can't even remember the secret! When I finally get it right, I want to sing the *Hallelujah Chorus*!

One of Scott's involuntary hide and seek adventures occurred on a rainy, autumn night while he was a youth pastor. While sitting at the top of the bleachers at a Holly High School Friday night football game, Scott whimsically decided to remove his wedding ring.

"Absence makes the heart grow fonder."
·- American proverb

"Oh, no!" Scott yelled. "My wedding ring! It's gone!" Evidently, the ring had fallen 40 feet below, into a muddy mess. Like any quick-thinking husband would do, he approached the announcer and requested that this message be given immediately over the sound system: "A wedding ring has been lost here tonight. It's somewhere under the bleachers. The person who finds it will be given $20 right away." All of a sudden, a slew of children crawled out of the bleachers and mingled in the muddy mess (much to the dismay of the moms who were present!) Sure enough, one pre-teen boy, caked in mud, approached Scott and demanded (as if he were Spider Man or James Bond), "Tell me what it looks like!" Scott replied, "It's gold, and it's round!" Sounding like a gangster himself, he continued, "Come on, kid – give me the ring, and I'll give you the dough!"

Fortunately that ring is still on Scott's finger. More important than the ring, however, are the commitment and the anticipation of our future together. If our search in life is only for temporal things, how shallow is that search? But when we set our heart, our affections, and our anticipations on what's above, then this life on earth suddenly takes on a whole new meaning.

"The place where your treasure is, is the place you will most want to be, and end up being."
~ Luke 12:34 (The Message)

How do you play hide and seek? Often the degree to which an item is considered lost depends upon its value. What do you value in life? Are your treasures on earth or in heaven? Keep your eye on the prize that does not perish, and don't give up the hunt!

"Before beginning a hunt, it is wise to ask someone what you are looking for before you begin looking for it."
~ Winnie the Pooh

Happy New Year

"Youth is when you're allowed to stay up late on New Year's Eve. Middle age is when you're forced to."
~ Bill Vaughn

New Years' Day is the most globally anticipated day of the year. Why is that? People put the past behind them and embrace the new. New Year's Day defies all barriers of culture, country, creed, religion, language, race, and age. Young children anticipate actually staying up past midnight, *with permission.* Strangers kiss. Horns blow. Prayers are said while lights glow. Balls fall. Balloons rise. A new calendar starts. Expectations sky.

What kind of expectations do you have for yourself at the New Year?

"I've always got such high expectations for myself. I'm aware of them, but I can't relax them."
~ Mary Decker Stanley

Expectations can be realized when we set realistic goals. When you hear the word "goals," what comes to your mind? Do you think of boundaries and borders? I think of open spaces and creative places. Goals and I are like bosom buddies. Just the sight of the word sparks a fire in my bones. This was quite evident when, with the deepest of high school convictions, I asked my close buddy, "Inger…what are your goals for Christmas vacation?" I fully admired her for her candid response: "Lisa, I don't have any goals over Christmas vacation! That's why they call it a *vacation!*"

What's so noble about setting goals?

Experts tell us:

"You don't have to be a fantastic hero to do certain things to compete. You can be just an ordinary chap, sufficiently motivated to reach challenging goals."
~ Edmund Hillary - Mount Everest conqueror

"Give me a stock clerk with a goal and I'll give you a man who will make history. Give me a man with no goals and I'll give you a stock clerk."
~ J.C. Penney

"If you're bored with life – you don't get up every morning with a burning desire to do things – you don't have enough goals."
~ Lou Holtz - Legendary Notre Dame football coach

Do you quiver when you read the word "goal"? Let me put you at ease. It's a four-letter word with life-changing opportunities. My eighth grade science teacher, Dr. Ackley, required us to write down our weekly goals in four major areas: physical, spiritual, social, and intellectual.

I can't explain how those goals helped me comprehend mass or distance, but they definitely expanded my understanding of "work." Work was defined as force times distance; if I wanted to accomplish my daily dreams or yearly aspirations, I had to take my own mass and move it a distance! Sitting still would do me no good.

"If you want to conquer fear, don't sit at home and think about it. Go out and get busy."
~ Dale Carnegie

"What are your goals now, Lisa?" you might gently jab. My goal for the New Year (which can start any day in one's heart) is to finish this book and finish it well. Is this goal realistic? Yes. Is it measurable? Of course – it's in your hand in black and white. Is this goal mine or is this someone else's goal for me? I completely own this goal. When my author friend and Personal Value Coaching President Maryanna Young wrote, "Do you have a book inside of you?" I felt like she knew me from the inside out. I've aspired to write a book for at least 30 years.

How about you? Try writing down your goals. Find a friend to keep you accountable and anticipate the exceptional life you've always dreamed of. Happy New Year's Day…today!

Moving the Tassel

Guest Author: Autumn M. Harper

To illustrate the anticipation of high school graduation, I've asked my oldest daughter Autumn, a graduating senior, to share her insights for parents, in particular. Autumn's experiences are indicative of many graduating high school seniors today.

> *"You have brains in your head.*
> *You have feet in your shoes. You can steer yourself*
> *in any direction you choose. You're on your own.*
> *And you know what you know.*
> *You are the guy who'll decide where to go."*
> ~ Dr. Seuss

When I was a little girl, I enjoyed asking my parents questions with obvious answers. As a young know-it-all, it gave me a sort of satisfaction to already know what would be coming out of their mouths. In fact, I was often very straightforward with my interrogating. "Daddy, when I turn 18, will you kick me out of the house?" Of course I knew what the answer would be from my loving father, but his response was different than my eight-year-old mind expected: "Of course we won't throw you out into the cold." I grinned smugly. "But there will be new expectations for you once you graduate!"

Along with new expectations from my parents come the questions. "Are you excited to graduate?" I can't even count how many times I have heard this my senior and even junior year. Sometimes I say no, sometimes I say yes, and when I can't think of anything to say, I laugh with uncertainty. My answer varies from day to day, because it's not a simple answer for me. I view the anticipation of my graduation not only as a one-hour event at Eastern Michigan University (consisting of 500 of my fellow peers), but also as the next mile stretch in my marathon of life. Why do I look at graduation this way? I consider this the point when I turn from a somewhat naïve teenager to a responsible, college-bound adult. That's a lot of pressure for a senior to swallow in one afternoon!

So how did my parents help prepare me for graduation? Thankfully, my parents have given me the opportunity to make difficult choices, whether I have wanted to or not. Not until recently have I realized how rare my upbringing has been in this aspect. For example, my schooling has taken many turns. I have gone from being home schooled to attending a small Christian school to attending a public high school campus, Plymouth-Canton Educational Park, with 6,000 diverse students. I ultimately decided all of these choices, with my parents' support. Their hope kindled my dreams, fueling a new courage within me.

141

"I hope your dreams take you to the corners of your smiles, to the highest of your hopes, to the windows of your opportunities, and to the most special places your heart has ever known."
~ Anonymous

What is there to anticipate? I look forward to studying music (and perhaps psychology) in college and making more daily decisions on my own. Whether I attend a public university twenty minutes from my home or a Christian university 1,000 miles away, I know that my parents have prepared me well. God will help me. On a practical note, I also look forward to taking classes later in the day, rather than having my first class start at 7 AM like it does at Salem High School. (Having such early classes has given me a new appreciation for parents who go to work in the morning while it's still dark outside!)

"I think sleeping was my problem in school. If school had started at 4 in the afternoon, I'd be a college graduate today."
~ George Foreman

I guess there's something special about the graduating ceremony after all. Although the diploma I will receive will just be in the temporary form of an empty tube until the authentic one arrives in the mail, I'm anticipating feeling the burden of four years of education lifted at that moment. Moving the tassel from right to left and tossing my cap is certainly a tradition I'm looking forward to, symbolizing the finish line in the race of my high school education. As far as living on my own goes, even though I still need to learn how to cook and balance my checkbook, at least I know how to do my laundry!

Question from Lisa: If you are a parent or a parental figure, how can you best equip your children for the graduations in life?

STAGE 8

Celebration

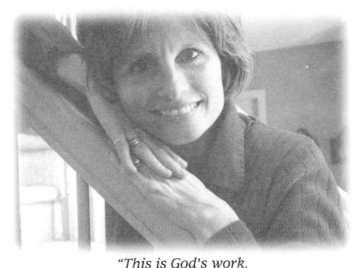

"This is God's work.
We rub our eyes—we can hardly believe it!
This is the very day God acted—
Let's celebrate and be festive!"

(The Message)

Celebrating the Marathon of Life

*H*ow do you celebrate when you have just coura-geously tackled an astounding challenge? Do you go out to eat? See a movie? Enjoy a bowl of ice cream? Golf 18 holes? Take a picture? Call a friend? Catch a nap? Watch more football? Text a buddy? Write thank-you notes? Plan a vacation? Crank up the stereo? Paint a picture? Go for a walk? Update your Facebook? Whistle a happy tune?

> *Happy days are here again.*
> *The skies above are clear again.*
> *Let us sing a song of cheer again.*
> *Happy days are here again!*
> ~ Jack Yellen

When I finish a marathon I have almost the same sense of accomplishment as going through child labor. To illustrate, when I was in lengthy labor (48 hours) with my daughter Autumn, I told myself, "Lisa, you ran that hard marathon (3:09) in 1985. If you can run a marathon, you can get through this!

> *"If God sends us on strong paths,*
> *we are provided with strong shoes."*
> ~ Corrie TenBoom

Do you know what I told myself after all of our children were born, when I decided to run that 2002 Detroit marathon with six days notice? (Keep in mind that it had been 17 years since I ran a marathon, and I never thought I would do another one again.) "Lisa, you went through all of those hard labors (four kids and five miscarriages). If you can do *that*, then you can run this marathon!" Thus, my first marathon prepared me for the mental and physical rigors of childbirth, and all of the childbirths prepared me well for the nine marathons since then! To me, this is cause for celebration!

"We are different, in essence, from other men.
If you want to win something, run 100 meters.
If you want to experience something,
run a marathon."
~ Emil Zatopek

How do I celebrate the completion of my marathons? After I take a hot bath, I talk to close family and friends on the phone as well as replay the marathon in detail with my running husband, Scott. I also treat myself to a piece of carrot cake. Well, I should clarify: I treat myself to the thick, butter cream frosting on the cake. The cake itself I could do without. Finally, I celebrate by typing out my marathon reflections, before the special effects of the moment leave my memory. Senior moments are common after my marathons! (Some of these marathon memories are included in my Marathon Mission blog at www.marathonmission.net.)

"Either write something worth reading
or do something worth writing."
~ Benjamin Franklin

Physically speaking, I sleep like a baby the night after a marathon. Or I should say that I sleep like a statue, because the slightest movement hurts and wakes me up. Furthermore, my leg muscles are full of lactic acid; walking up and down steps looks like I've got wooden legs. Light stretching and massages always help. Lastly, I enjoy the freedom of taking the next week off from running. Gentle walks, arm in arm with my Honey, are my remedy for recovery!

"He who limps is still walking."
~ Stanislaw J. Lec

Your life is like a marathon, too. Will you ponder on the sequence of these events: inspiration, preparation, perspiration, initiation, continuation, obstruction, anticipation, and celebration? Now linger a little longer on that last word…celebration. Go ahead…celebrate your triumphs with gusto. Just remember to tell people where your help comes from!

*"I lift up my eyes to the hills - where does my
help come from? My help comes from the Lord,
Maker of heaven and earth!"*

~ Psalm 21:1, 2 (NIV)

Kudos for Character

"If friends were flowers, I'd pick you."
~ Anonymous

Celebrate friendship! While those two words might sound a little cheesy or cliché, they are actually quite powerful when placed together. According to Webster's Thesaurus, "celebrate" has numerous lively synonyms:

> *Celebrate v. –" To give indulgence to a celebration; feast, give a party, rejoice, kill the fatted calf, go on a spree, revel, blow off steam, let off steam, have a party, have a ball, kick up one's heels, let loose, let go, live it up, whoop it up, make merry, party."*

Is it just me, or is it easier to celebrate with a friend than alone? (When have you had a party all alone? Pity parties don't count!)

A true friend is dependable, loyal, and forgiving. Friendship is also a two way street, not so much a give and a take, but a give and a give! I'm ashamed of an occasion in elementary school when I was anything but friendly. Two of us girls on the Gesu school bus wanted to play with the "popular girl" Joanna. Like any predictable, self-centered catfight among girls, both of us literally held on to each one of Joanna's arms and played tug of war on the bus with her body! "You're coming to MY house," I tugged. "No, you're coming to MY house," yanked the other catwoman. This went on for several minutes when I finally realized that this was not the way to get a friend or treat a friend. So I let go. That was a turning point for me in my friendships. I looked into the mirror of selfishness, and didn't like what I saw. No more gossip and games for me. God changed me from the inside out.

True friendship is worth celebrating, and too many of us wait until our friends die to tell them how much we love them. Who are some of your closest friends? When was the last time you told them something about their character that you appreciate? The Harper family has a tradition of doing this on birthdays. We individually share "kudos for character" with the birthday person. The birthday person often shares affirmative words in return; it's a marvelous exchange of kindness!

"My best friend is the one who
brings out the best in me."
~ Henry Ford

Which friends bring out the best in you? How do they do this? As an adolescent I learned of the Proverb, "He who has friends must himself be friendly." That shocked me a bit. If I were not intentionally friendly, then I would not have friends. Friendliness is not just for kids, it's for adults, too. In fact, we could learn a lesson or two from them.

"My father always used to say that when you die,
if you've got five real friends,
then you've had a great life."
~ Lee Iacocca

I celebrate the longevity of these friendships:

Reneé, Cathy, Inger, Wendy, Julie, Lizzi, and
Frances…I've known you for 30 years and over.
Becky, Christine, Maryanna, Laura, Chris,
Lori, and Sue…can we visit on a layover?
Georgette, Carol, Criss, Cindy, Edie, and
Theresa…you serve with such devotion.
Nancy, Christina, Josie, Judy, Barb, and
Donna…giving in perpetual motion.
Vivian, Kim, Lisa, Holly, Rosie, and Erin…
you make music anywhere.
Diane, Brenda, Joan, Jenny, Katherine, June,
and Kathi…thanks for the ways you care.
Dorothy, Judy, Nancy, Marilyn, and Silvia…
pastor's wives whom I admire.
Marlene, Terrie, Mayra, Dawn, Helen, Heather,
and Patricia…you're a stitch… how you inspire!

These friends have been with me through thick and thin, and the list is far from complete. Do you appreciate such devotion in your friends as well? If so, try the "kudos for character" on for size...and celebrate your friendships!

Laugh Out Loud

"A person without a sense of humor
is like a wagon without springs,
jolted by every pebble in the road."
~ Henry Ward Beecher

When was the last time you laughed? I mean, really laughed? Laughter and celebration often go hand-in-hand. Not only do I want to live my life out loud (as an outward expression of the inward work God continually does in me) but I want to laugh out loud, too. I'll be the first one to admit that I need to do it more often.

What are the benefits of laughter? According to *Alternative Therapies of Health and Medicine,* there exist a myriad of advantages of laughter as they relate to stress management. Laughter strengthens the immune system by increasing certain healthy hormones. It can distract us from anger (when necessary) and other tough emotions. In addition, laughter provides a physical or emotional release, giving us a better perspective on life. What happens to you when someone in the room starts laughing? Sooner or later, you will probably start laughing too, because laughter is contagious! Laughter is also free and convenient.

"Laughter is an instant vacation."

~ Anonymous

Our family always laughs when we watch the acclaimed *I Love Lucy* reruns. In one hilarious show, Lucille Ball stuffs hordes of chocolates into her mouth all in an attempt to keep up with the ever-increasing speed of a factory's conveyor belt full of bon bons. I call this "humor therapy!" Actually, when my kids are sick or sad, we often play *I Love Lucies*. (Proverbs even tells us that "a merry heart is like a medicine!") For a brief moment, their worries disappear in the thralls of belly-busting laughter.

Kids say the darndest things. When one of my children started growing taller than me, she asked with all seriousness, "Mommy, are you done growing?" "Yes," I answered. "Really?" she questioned with deep empathy. "Oh...I'm sorry. Are you a dork?" At that moment I burst out laughing. Then I had to reign myself in, because my sprouting daughter was completely soberminded. She had meant, "dwarf." I reassured her, "You don't have to feel sorry for me for being short. God has a plan for me to be a short mom. God has a plan for you to be a taller girl. I'm okay with that honey, and you can be too!"

As a parent, these innocent comments by other children (www.rinksworks.com) make me laugh out loud. How about you?

"When I go to heaven, I want to see my grandpa again. But he better have lost the nose hair and the old-man smell."
– Age 5

"Don't kid me, Mom, I know they're my feet."
– 3-year-old son, when his mother told him his shoes were on the wrong feet

"And lead us not into temptation, but deliver us some email."
– 4-year-old girl, misquoting the Lord's Prayer

"When your mom is mad at your dad, don't let her brush your hair."
– Morgan, age 11

"One of you should know how to write a check, because even if you have tons of love, there is still going to be a lot of bills."
– Ava, age 8, when asked what she thought about love and marriage

"Daddy, did your hair slip?"
– 3-year-old son, to his bald but long bearded father

"Tell me when you're asleep, okay?"
– 7-year-old son, overheard talking to his 5 year old brother.

These days are serious enough. Will you join with me in celebrating life…with laughter? Find a friend who lightens your load (like my high school pal Reneé does for me, over a cup of chai tea. Or Scott's brothers do for him while watching a lively sporting event.) Put your burdens on the shelf for a moment (or better yet, in God's hands forever)…and laugh out loud! If we can do it, so can you!

Mutual Celebration Society

"Welcome every morning with a smile...
You were not born to fail."
~ Og Mandino

"Mommy, why won't God let me fly?" As an inquisitive preschooler, I had tearfully sauntered up to my mom's Queen Anne's chair and tugged on her skirt for some heart-to-heart advice.

Mommy, I really want to fly! I told God that I would not believe in Him unless He let me fly. I've been trying all morning. I went on the first step and flapped my arms like a bird. Then I jumped off, and it didn't work. I didn't fly. I fell down. I kept trying this all the way up to step four. Momma, I don't understand, because I know that God is real, so I thought by now He would let me fly. Plus, I don't think He wants me to keep falling down like this. It hurts when I fall down, especially when I go higher. I can't do it anymore. Mommy, why won't God let me fly?

With all of the wisdom of a well-seasoned veteran, my mother replied, "Honey, if God wanted you to fly, He would have made you a bird." Hmmm...I had to think about that for a minute. Then it made perfectly good sense. God didn't make me a bird. He made me a little girl. Although I was disappointed in His non-flight decision, God knew what was best when He created me. Fine by me! Wouldn't it be great if we all continued to trust God with the simple faith of a child?

Not long after that I proceeded to ask my good-hearted mother another philosophical preschool question: "Mommy, do you love God more than me?" Can you guess what she said? What would you have answered? She replied, "Yes, Sweetheart, I do!" Some children may have been crushed by this answer; I was not. Quite the contrary. "Wow," I reasoned. "I know mom loves me a lot, so she must *really* love God!"

Therein were my first memories of God and His love. What a reason to celebrate! Looking back on your life, can you identify times when God has been with you? Remember the old movie, *It's a Wonderful Life*? George (Jimmy Stewart) got a glimpse into what life would have been like all around him if he weren't alive. Confusion, selfishness, anger, and discontent were rampant.

"You've been given a great gift, George: A chance to see what the world would be like without you."
~ Clarence, the Angel in *It's a Wonderful Life*

How much more would your life and mine be altered without God in our lives? All of mankind is born with a figurative "whole in the heart" that only God can fill.

We search for fulfillment in all sorts of empty places: relationships, material goods, sports, children, promotions, influence, looks, status, degrees, fame, wealth, popularity, acceptance (and even running, if it becomes an idol). Gratefully, we can come to God as we are, warts and all. He knit us together in our mother's womb (Psalm 139), and He longs for us to draw close, like I did to my mother's hem.

"God smiled the day you were born!"
~ Anonymous

I hereby declare a Mutual Celebration Society! God celebrates the lives of us, and we celebrate a life full of Him!

How do we celebrate a life full of God? We can't fly by flapping our arms and jumping off house steps, but we sure can soar in even better ways.

"They that wait upon the Lord shall renew
their strength; They shall mount up with wings
as eagles; They shall run, and not be weary;
and they shall walk, and not faint."
~ Isaiah 40:31

Living Out Loud

"If you ask me what I came to do in this world,
I, an artist, will answer you:
I am here to live out loud."

~ Emile Zola

*I*t is finished! This book is finished! Today I celebrate. Going from "blank to book" has been a remarkable journey.

When you have a personal goal, do you tell your world about it or keep it to yourself? I kept my book-writing goal a relative secret. Why? I only wanted to hear, "That a girl!" and not, "You can't write a book!"

"This writing business. Pencils and what-not.
Over-rated, if you ask me. Silly stuff. Nothing in it."

~ Eeyore

Who do you share your dreams with? Purposely pursue positive people. Keep your hand to the plow with the end in sight, and get ready to celebrate with all your might! My plow involved writing almost every day: pre-writing, writing, revising, editing, and sharing the draft. While sometimes intimidating to sit down in front of an empty computer screen, I welcomed the new challenge.

"Exercise the writing muscle every day, even if it is only a letter, notes, a title list, a character sketch, a journal entry. Writers are like dancers, like athletes. Without that exercise, the muscles seize up."

~ Jane Yolen

What helps you think creatively and live out loud? When I run, I always think creatively. Thus, while writing each story in this book, I would run before, during, or after the daily drafting. Do you know one of my creative ideas that came to me while running? I envisioned typing on my computer while running on my treadmill! Can you imagine the creative juices that would flow if I were given the opportunity to write and run at the same time? Never say never!

I would be remiss if I did not mention the hardest parts in writing this book, for I've heard that the greatness of the victory is often determined by the greatness of the struggle. "Cut. Cut. Cut!" I found editing to be particularly painful, because I love words.

Want to know a secret? There were a few times when I sat at my computer and faced significant unexpected hurdles. For example, the day before my final book deadline, which entailed emailing this entire book to my interior designer, my Internet server malfunctioned. My printer also refused to print. The very next morning our roof had a leak. Water dripped down the inside walls of our house from top to bottom, seeping through our basement ceiling and right onto our computer desk! (Reminder: *Living and Loving* was stored in that computer!) Frankly, I was in no mood to be electrocuted. I had been preparing to celebrate. Of all the places in the entire house that water could have fallen from the ceiling, it happened to fall right onto the *computer!* In addition, on a few previous writing occasions, somehow what I had just typed onto the computer screen was erased into thin air. I must have clicked the wrong "X"!

How do you respond when you get the wind knocked out of your sails? At that "vanishing word" moment, I dug deep into my core, making this faith declaration: "Lord, you promise that you work all things together for my good (Romans 8:28), so I choose to trust you now. I dare to believe that the second draft can be even better than the first. With fortitude and joy, I will take a dose of my own hope-filled medicine and persevere. Blue skies are coming."

> *"In my experience, the best creative work is never done when one is unhappy."*
> ~ Albert Einstein

Some celebrations are quite festive and public. While I may experience a bit of that on my "book opening day", the greatest satisfaction of "living out loud" will happen in the quietness of my heart, when I place a copy of this book into each of my children's memory boxes. Someday they will read this and remember when their mama faced the unexplored mountain of book writing. With God's help, she made it to the summit. They can too. So can you!

Whatever challenges you face in your marathon of life, with God as your Guide, you too, can scale your mountain, one step at a time. By the way, once you've reached your summit, make sure you give God some praise and *celebrate out loud!*

About Lisa M. Harper

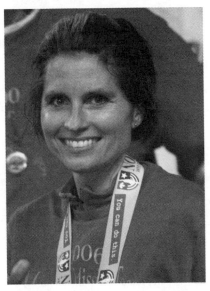

*I*n two words: *Irresistible force.* That's how friends describe Lisa M. Harper – a motivator, encourager, and worker whose zest for living is nothing short of contagious. Motivating others to achieve their "unattainable" dreams, while empathizing with their struggles, Harper offers her friends a unique blend of reflection, compassion and inspiration. Although Harper has rarely met a challenge she couldn't overcome, her life experiences include setbacks, heartaches, *and* losses women and men can identify with. However, as Harper has discovered and now shares, that although circumstances do play a role, many times a person's greatest challenge and obstacle in life is really just himself or herself. Sometimes people lack the confidence to even take a step…much less an entirely new (running) route in life. Harper's candid insights and positive faith inspire others to experience the electricity of life while fulfilling their God-given destiny.

Lisa M. Harper earned her Masters of Arts degree from Eastern Michigan University and resides in the Detroit, Michigan area. As an active pastor's wife, soccer mom, educator, speaker, musician, runner, Marathon Mission founder and author, Lisa is *Living and Loving – The Marathon of Life*.

To contact Lisa for speaking engagements, email her at lisa@marathonmission.net or call 734.775.3073.

DIGGING DEEPER INTO YOUR
Living and Loving –The Marathon of Life
STUDY

Many of you have requested a list of Bible verses to go along with *Living and Loving – The Marathon of Life.* Here are just a few. Enjoy your digging!

INSPIRATION

- Ephesians 1:3,4
- Ephesians 3:20-21
- Isaiah 40:27-32
- Philippians 4:13
- Romans 8:18-21

PREPARATION

- II Peter 3:14
- II Timothy 2:2
- Ephesians 4:11-13
- Proverbs 13:4
- Matthew 13:18-23

PERSPIRATION

- Romans 8:18-21
- James 1:12
- II Corinthians 4:7-11
- Romans 8:28
- Matthew 7:7-11

INITIATION
- Philippians 1:6
- Mark 3:13-15
- II Timothy 1:6,9
- Psalm 71:14-16
- Psalm 111:10

CONTINUATION
- James 1:12
- II Timothy 1:6,9
- Psalm 146:1,2
- James 1:22
- Colossians 1:10

OBSTRUCTION
- Romans 5:1-5
- Psalm 42:11
- Romans 8:31-39
- John 16:33
- II Timothy 2:1-15

ANTICIPATION
- Ephesians 3:20
- Hebrews 12:1,2
- Jeremiah 29:11-13
- Ephesians 1:15-21
- Philippians 3:12-15

CELEBRATION
- Psalm 100
- Psalm 103:1-5
- Psalm 118:21-25
- Psalm 126
- Psalm 150

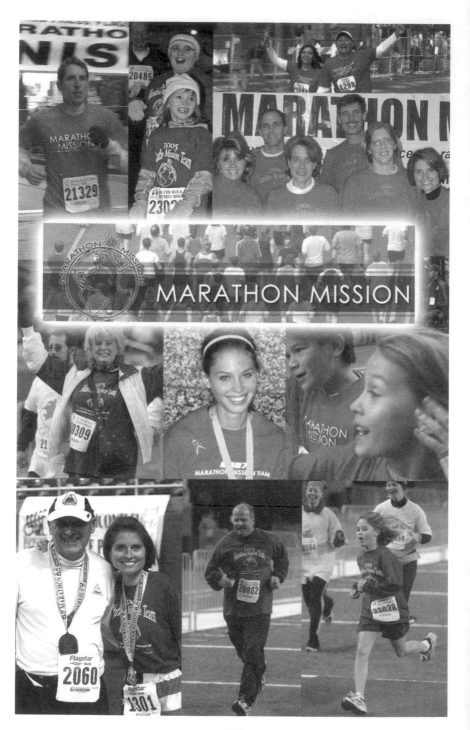

MARATHON MISSION

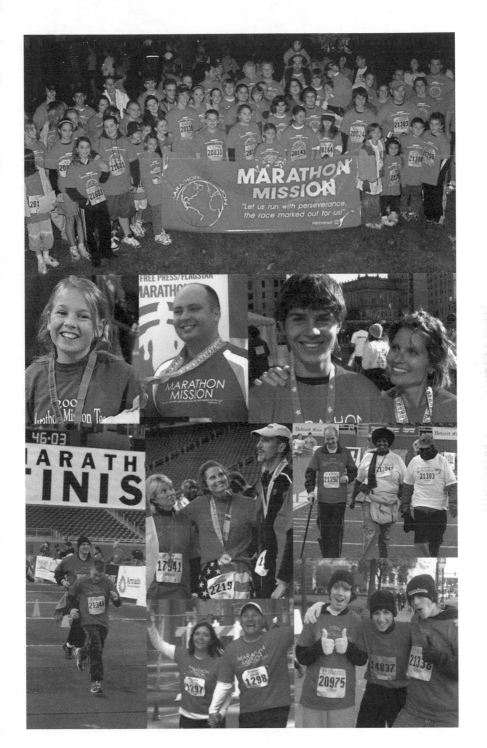

*M*arathon Mission founder, Lisa M. Harper, has taken two meaningful areas of everyday living and combined them into one life-changing cause: Marathon Mission. These two components are health and compassion. The 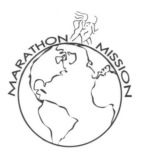 Marathon Mission team remains physically active while loving our neighbor. Today you can take these components and make positive strides in your health and the vitality of the world around you when you join the Marathon Mission team. Our team is made up of participants, volunteers, supporters and charity leaders.

Marathon Mission began in 2003 with one lone marathon runner, Lisa M. Harper, running her 26.2 miles with the Detroit Free Press/Flagstar Marathon. The news spread quickly. More and more walkers and runners were inspired to use their strength for a reason beyond themselves. Incorporated in 2006, Marathon Mission now gathers a multitude of walkers and runners to participate in marathons and other racing events nation wide. Marathon Mission team participants of all ages and abilities walk or jog various distances to raise financial support for dozens of worthy charitable organizations and non-profit corporations.

Usually 100% of the funds raised go directly to causes such as these (including Marathon Mission itself):

Autism Research Institute
Beat the Odds
Bless India Ministries
Boys and Girls Missionary
  Crusade
Budapest Care Center
Carrie and Matt Love
Chi Alpha – Eastern
  Michigan University
Coates Ministries of Kenya
City Mission
Coins for Kids
Youth for Christ- Cleveland
Convoy of Hope
Cure SMA for Erinne
Dearborn Assembly of God
First Assembly Food Bank
Fowlerville Freedom Center
Heroes of the Faith Missions
Hillcrest Orphanage
In Memory of Amy Lyzenga
India Missions
Joy of Jesus
Jamaica Christian School
  for the Deaf
King of Love University
  Church

Latino Christian Center
MAPS to Argentina
Michigan Missions/Church
  Plants
Obadiah Ministries
Mission Aviation Fellowship
Neighborhood Legal Services
ONEWAY Youth
Open Arms Lutheran Church
Oral Roberts University
MM ORU Scholarship
Possessing the Land-
  Connection Church
Promise Village
Seeds of Faith
Robin's Nest Children's
  Home
Southfield Christian School
Speed the Light
Speers Family- Mexico
The Navigators
Unlimited Vision/ WM'S
Wellspring
Wycliffe Bible Translators
Younglife/Wyldlife

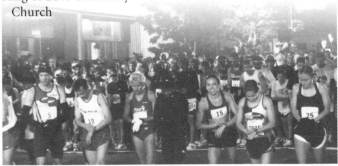

- Visit www.marathonmission.net to see how you can do Marathon Mission in Detroit or in your neck of the woods!

- At www.marathonmission.net you will find a host of helpful tools to make your Marathon Mission experience both meaningful and rewarding.

- Tour our stimulating photos, video footage, helpful packets, pledge sheets, support letters, colorful flyers and more.

- Email one of our expert, on-line Marathon Mission trainers for just the advice you need.

- Visit their blogs as well as Lisa Harper's blog for the latest thoughts on what makes them tick and how you can reach your potential, too!

- Drop Lisa an email anytime! She would love to hear what fuels your fire! Lisa@marathonmission.net

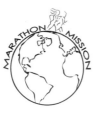

MARATHON MISSION
You really CAN do this!
Marathon Mission
PO Box 262
Clare, MI 48617
Phone: 734.775.3073
www.marathonmission.net

Acknowledgements

*I*am told that recognizing individuals for their assistance is like a minefield. I will surely forget to say thank you to someone. Nevertheless, I am one to take risks in this department. I think it's well worth it!

All successful projects in life take team effort. *Living and Loving – The Marathon of Life* is no different.

It's important to give honor to whom honor is due. My heartfelt gratitude is extended to the following:

Maryanna Young – You were the first one who sparked my author's heart when you wrote, "Is there a book inside of you?" Yes, there is. Through your friendship and guidance you've helped make my authoring path straight. I strongly recommend your book, *From Book to Blank…From Idea to Amazon in 150 Days*, to any prospective author.

Dan and Lori Van Veen – Your editing advice is supreme, not to mention your top-notch friendship skills. Our prewriting brainstorming during our Marathon Mission 2008 weekend was a turning point for the direction of this book. Thank you for believing in me and for your countless hours of correspondence.

Church staff and families at Bethesda Christian Church, Davisburg Methodist Church, Mt. Bethel Church, The Shores Church (St. Clair Shores Assembly of God and Powerhouse), Hope Alive Assembly, First Assembly of God, Connection Church and Clare Assembly of God. Thanks for allowing me to be so involved in the fabric of your congregations. I cherish you. Leading and serving with you have made me who I am.

Assemblies of God Michigan District staff, including Bill and Marilyn Leach, Jeff Kennedy, Steve Bradshaw, Mary Selzer, and Trudy Grenier – You have dealt very well with my zealous ways and big Marathon Mission ideas, particularly with Speed the Light, BGMC, Home and Foreign Missions, Women's Ministry (Unlimited Vision), Chi Alpha, and Church Planting. Thanks for the continued opportunities and support.

Southfield Christian School, Dr. Hall, Dr. Ackley, Doug Olsen, and staff – You skillfully trained me to passionately pursue excellence for the glory of God. In my book, you are the premier Christian school in Michigan. Go SCS!

Borgo School of Dance and Gymnastics: Frances, Virginia, and staff – I spent ten wonderful years learning from you. You taught me how to envision myself as a winner and hold my head up high, with the unique blend of manners, humility, confidence, and character.

Joy of Jesus, the late founder Rev. Eddie Edwards, Mary Edwards, and current president, Allen Sheffield – As a teenager you believed in me enough to allow me to counsel other young people in need. You taught me the strength of giving a hand up, not just a hand out. My model of service and ministry started with J of J.

Oral Roberts and Oral Roberts University students, alumni and staff – My days on the ORU campus were some of the best years of my life. Thank you, Oral, for training up your students to hear God's voice. I now go where God's voice is heard small, His light is dim, and His healing power is not known. I do expect a miracle. I also believe that God is my Source and that something good is going to happen to us today.

Marathon Mission board (Tim, Allen, Jeffrey, Anton), bookkeeper (Brenda), office assistants (Josie and Kathi), videographer (Tom), photographers (Jeff, Rosie, and Katie), volunteers (Carol, Jenn, Mick, Russ, and many more), participants, supporters, and charity heads – You are like my second family. Many of you have been cheering me on to write this book. I appreciate your belief in me and better yet, your commitment to joining me as we use our strength to make an enduring impact for all things God!

Patricia Ball – You were the first Marathon Director (Detroit Free Press/Flagstar Marathon) in the United States to welcome Marathon Mission into the official fold of worthy reasons to run or walk. You've got a heart of gold and are a true champion yourself.

Detroit Free Press/Flagstar Marathon staff – You have been exceedingly kind to me as the director of Marathon Mission and always gracious with the Marathon Mission team. Thank you.

Friends of Lisa – I would not be the same without the listening ears, pats on the back, gentle prodding (and gifts of chocolate) throughout the years. From my childhood friends to college roommates to neighbors to fellow moms, your friendship is a priceless treasure.

Families Galore: Hutchens, Matsons, Brokos, Kiefts, Woods, Dewars, Hunts, Cordinas, Campbells, Falgetellis, Coates, Andresses, Thompsons, Distads, all First Assembly Families, all Connection Families – What a joy to raise our families at the same time.

Principals and staff at Field Elementary, East Middle School, and Plymouth-Canton Educational Park – Thank you for partnering with our family in bringing outstanding education to the Harper children.

Dr. Eduardo Garcia and staff – You have supported me through nine pregnancies and constantly challenged me to have hope.

Anna, Matthew, Breanna, and Sean – You keep me running in life and current with the Facebook times.

Katie Kieft, Tom Martindale, and Jeff Kindy – The pictures in this book never would have happened without you.

Tim, Donna, Kathy, Julie, Diane, Maryanna, Autumn, and Mark Anthony – Your proof reading skills were a tremendous asset to me.

Woodcreek friends – You have witnessed me run in all kinds of conditions (and outfits)! Thank you for your waves of affirmation for over a decade.

RECESS: Heather Gneco, Christy McDonald, teachers and families – My family loved being part of your homeschool co-op for seven growth-filled years.

My father and step-mother, Tom and Kathy Nutt; My mother and step-father, Donna Cummings and Rick Donovan; My mother-in-law, Anne Harper – Each one of you brings a needed perspective into my life. I love you all.

Nutt extended family: Aunt Mary Lou and Uncle Harold, Aunt Doris and Uncle Frank, Aunt Del and

Uncle John, Aunt Therese and Uncle Pat, Aunt Cathy and Uncle Chuck, Aunt Carole and Uncle Art, Uncle Mel, Uncle Mike, and dozens of cousins – I inherited my tireless work ethic from you. Can one of you take me on a vacation?

Perlich family: Aunt Pat, Uncle Francis (Mickey) and Aunt Pam, Aunt Carolyn, Aunt Louise and Uncle Dennis, and cousins – You have always showered me with love and laughter.

Harper extended family: Clark, Fred, Mark, Deborah, Mark Jr., Katherine, Missy, and the Winsor family – Thanks for your lives of hope, dedication and generosity.

Tim and Marlene Cummings – Your unconditional love and support throughout the years have been a pillar of fortitude and empowerment in my life.

My siblings and their spouses: Tom, Mark and Terrie, Julie and Mark William, Jeff and Mayra – Your commitment to God, family, and causes at hand motivate me to move mountains. I like being your baby sister.

To my immediate family: Scott, Autumn, Jonathan, Victoria, and Jasmine – You fill my days with purpose, liveliness, celebration, and exceptional living. You are my heroes. I cherish each day with you. We have seen as a family that with God, all things are possible. Together we are *Living and Loving – The Marathon of Life.*

"I don't know about you,
but I'm running hard for the finish line.
I'm giving it everything I've got.
No sloppy living for me!
I'm staying alert and in top condition.
I'm not going to get caught napping,
telling everyone else all about it
and then missing out myself."

(The Message)

"Pursue a righteous life:
a life of wonder, faith, love, steadiness, courtesy.
Run hard and fast in the faith.
Seize the eternal life, the life you were called to,
the life you so fervently embraced."

(The Message)

VerticalView Publishing
Quick Order Form

Available by Lisa M. Harper:

Living & Loving - The Marathon of Life
Experience the Electricity of Life!

Interspersing dozens of encouraging and thought-provoking quotes and quips throughout the pages, Harper's wit and wisdom will leave you softly laughing or quietly reflecting, but always deeply inspired $14.95

Postal Orders:
VerticalView Publishing, Lisa M. Harper
PO Box 262, Clare, MI 48617 USA

(Please send cashiers check or money order made out to: Lisa M. Harper)

Shipping and Handling:
$5.00 for first item and $2.00
for each additional item to same address.

Email Orders:
lisa@marathonmission.net

Online Orders:
www.themarathonoflife.com
Also available on Amazon.com

VerticalView Publishing
Quick Order Form

Available by Lisa M. Harper:

Living & Loving - The Marathon of Life
Experience the Electricity of Life!

Interspersing dozens of encouraging and thought-provoking quotes and quips throughout the pages, Harper's wit and wisdom will leave you softly laughing or quietly reflecting, but always deeply inspired $14.95

Postal Orders:
VerticalView Publishing, Lisa M. Harper
PO Box 262, Clare, MI 48617 USA

(Please send cashiers check or money order
made out to: Lisa M. Harper)

Shipping and Handling:
$5.00 for first item and $2.00
for each additional item to same address.

Email Orders:
lisa@marathonmission.net

Online Orders:
www.themarathonoflife.com
Also available on Amazon.com

MARATHON MISSION

You really CAN do this!

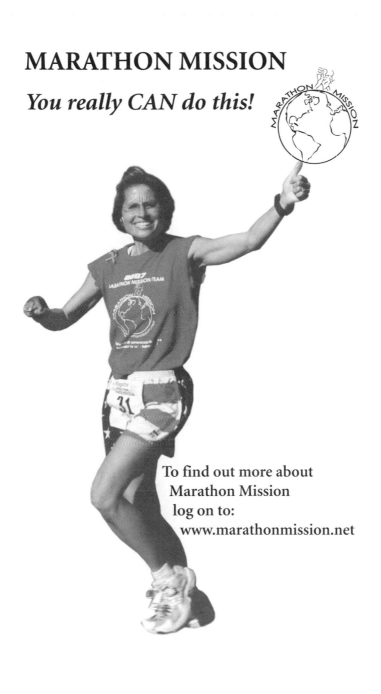

To find out more about
Marathon Mission
log on to:
www.marathonmission.net

"Trust God from the bottom of your heart;
don't try to figure out everything on your own.
Listen for God's voice in everything you do,
everywhere you go;
He's the one who will keep you on track.
Don't assume that you know it all.
Run to God!...Your body will glow with health.
Your very bones will vibrate with life!"

(The Message)